Personal Trainer Secrets
For Men Over 40

By

Jim Hart, A.C.E.

First published by AuthorHouse 05/13/04

ISBN: 1-4184-7346-4 (e-book)
ISBN: 1-4184-4154-6 (Paperback)

This book is printed on acid free paper.

- **Little known facts, 61 unusual tips, and effective shortcuts to getting the body you want**

- **Dozens of "Can't fail" strategies for getting lean and staying there**

- **Everything you need to know about cutting fat and adding muscle in the shortest time possible**

Jim Hart   –   Personal Trainer, A.C.E.
Physical Development Specialist
Lifestyle Coach
Master Chef

Edited by R Perry Monastero

The ultimate guide to fat burning & muscle building for the best years of your life

Table of Contents

Jim Hart's Training Philosophy

It's never too late to begin a fitness program and create the body you want. You should be able to feel good, healthy, and energized at any age. Exercise and healthy eating are choices that enhance the overall quality of life and can be fun and enjoyable as a daily activity. My program is a lifestyle choice, not a temporary quick fix weight loss gimmick. Being in my forties, I understand the physical and lifestyle issues men face as they age. I believe there are solutions to every issue related to the aging process.

I have the experience and wisdom from twenty years in the business of fitness and weight loss. I loss sixty pounds over twenty years ago and have maintained a low fat body. You can too! Through education and by example, I lead my clients on a journey of self-discovery, and have helped them create a new lifestyle of high energy, health, freedom from illness, a better mental and emotional outlook and tight, well-conditioned body.

book will help you to make the transition to the new road. And I'll help you to live the lifestyle in the body you've only dreamed about.

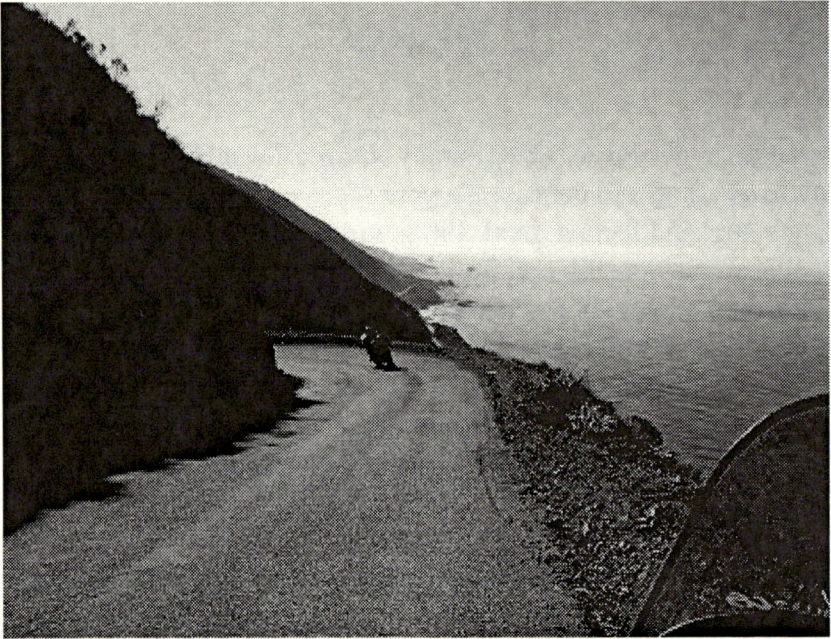

Who cares if you are sixty? I believe that age is no longer a barrier when it comes to having a muscular, lower fat body, with high-energy levels and outstanding health. Attitude plays a key role in the success of men in their prime years regarding fitness and weight loss goals. Your new outlook needs to be a mantra of *"Age is NOT a barrier"*. Your mental conditioning, as most men in our age group experienced, has been just the opposite. Once many of us hit forty, so often we feel programmed to believe that fitness, dreams and goals are foregone, that our body cannot look good, and that it's all over. Some call it "hitting the wall." Society's programming is reinforced though professional sports. Look at pro ball players retiring in their early thirties. Some say, "They're washed up, the body just can't take it any more!"

Right? I say ***WRONG***! The truth is, most pro sport athletes abuse and damage their bodies at extraordinarily super-high levels that most of us will never begin to know. Rather, you're probably like most men I train. Most men in their forties and older who have regular jobs are just beginning to reach their peak levels of strength and mental focus to make the changes necessary to maintain a role model body well into their sixties and beyond.

Come and run with me in my quest to help you gain a better body. Forget what you've tried in the past. Realize you can make a difference today. Starting with small incremental steps, I'll take you to the apex of fitness and to points where you never imagined you would go!

I do want you to try to have a sense of humor about your training as well. Here's an excerpt from an email sent from one trainee to another:

------ ---- ----- ----- ----- ----- ---- ----- ----- ----- ----- ----- ----- ----

Forwarded message:
Subj: Re: Cycle of Life
Date: 03/21/2002 9:40:06 PM Eastern Standard Time
From: Wburton999
To: VaughJCook

Dream on, Vaughnnie!

Just had a wonderful meal here at home that was great and under 500 calories! (I had eight strands of fettucini!)

I've discovered Jim's book is kind of like AA and drinking. You know how we say AA and all you learn about yourself and about alcohol ruins your drinking? Well, Jim Hart's book has ruined my unhealthy eating!

I hate her!

Bill

---- ----- ----- ----- ----- ---- ----- ----- ----- ----- ----- ----- ----- -----

Readers, I want you to know that you are free to contact me at any point during this program. By the way, you may visit my personal website or email me for advice, ideas, or motivation. I look forward to taking this personal journey with you

How to reach Jim Hart –
Visit the Hartbody website: http://www.hartbody.com
Email the author: hartbody@aol.com
Contact his gym: (12th Street Gym, Philadelphia) 215.985.4092

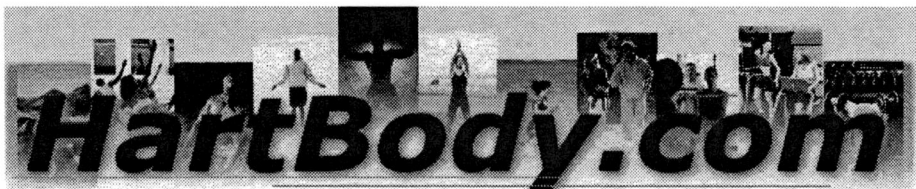

Tip #1: Don't buy into a negative aging mindset

Having energy to do the things you want to do now that you have the time and financial resources is of paramount importance. There is a new generation of Baby Boomers and those over sixty who are coming of age and continuing their fitness efforts. Many are enjoying active lifestyles while living longer, better quality lives. The key attitude to the new revolution I sometimes call the "Second Age" is this: the older you are, the more quality there should be in your levels of health and fitness. The Second Age can be the zenith of fitness for men over forty.

Many of us value "functionality," one key to living each day to its fullest. Possessing enough energy to walk up stairs without getting winded, lift heavy boxes without straining, and take long walks without tiring are key components of "functionality" as we age. Who wants to reach the apex of financial and career success and be stuck using a cane, walker, or wheelchair? Yet, many men who ignore exercise and good eating habits find themselves physically limited at a shockingly early age, while their exercising counterparts are running, playing tennis, and taking hiking vacations in the hill country of Tuscany. Get active now – don't miss out on the fun!

Despite all the good news about our fitness abilities in middle age, we still need to be cautious and compassionate with our bodies. As most aging athletes already know, our joints, muscles, and vital internal organs need extra care and attention if we are to keep them well-oiled and running at maximum efficiency throughout the length of our active lives. Our joints and muscles tell us when we're overdoing it and give us fair warnings through mild aches and pains. By stretching, resting, and following the techniques discussed later, you will understand how to maximize your longevity and maintain the look of muscular fitness and good health well into the advanced years.

When sidelined with a minor injury, there is no reason to cease playing sports, lifting weights, or doing aerobics. It's just part of the game and part of maturing gracefully. Sometimes an injury provides an opportunity to try different activities like yoga, Pilates, biking, hiking, swimming, karate, or Tae Bo. Plus, trying new activities makes life more fun and interesting.

As aging Baby Boomers, we experience some common physical and lifestyle changes. Sometimes our career, relationships, and self-perception (how we relate to the grand scheme of the world and our role in the great vegetable soup of life) are reevaluated in middle age. These mid-life passages drive us during the Second Age of life. The desire to do all we can increases as the realization that life is halfway over and the clock is ticking. Our lives accelerate, enriched with activities, adventures, and the burning desire to have all the things for which we've worked and struggled. Although our testosterone levels may gradually lower compared to our teens and twenties, our lust for life and its pleasures, both sensually and spiritually, are always present and in need of attention. How successful we are at integrating all the desires, goals, and fulfilling our dreams depends on how well we take care of our physical bodies. If we feel physically healthy, we can enjoy all that life offers us each and every fun-filled day.

Here's a wild thought: new advances in drugs and anti-aging medicine could make 100-years-old a new standard of longevity for men over the next thirty years. Many of us will live to that ripe old age in perfect health, enjoying fulfilling work, leisure activities, and healthy sexual relations. The future holds so much promise it would be foolish not to take control of our life now by exercising, eating right, and living a peaceful existence that supports happiness and fulfillment. Our lives can be ideal **if we work at it now**. Many of us may need to take advantage of the services of experts who can help us reach these goals. Personal trainers, nutritionists, anti-aging physicians, life coaches, personal chefs, and mental health professionals can help us to reach and maintain a long life of quality we never dreamed possible twenty years ago.

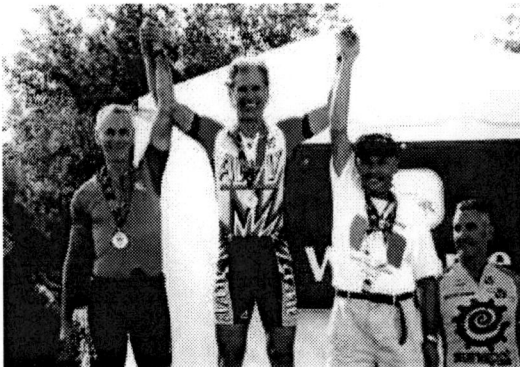

Nobody would deny that almost nothing is more valuable than time. Neither money nor material possessions will go with us into the afterlife. How we spend our time and the way we allocate it to living a life we love determines our level of happiness and how we feel physically, emotionally, mentally, socially, and spiritually. *Carpe diem* ("Seize the day") becomes more relevant as we age. Mortality is often a dirty word. Most of us don't think about death often, but we feel the reality when someone close to us is stricken with a fatal illness or a parent dies suddenly. I believe that life gives us reminders that can be used to a positive end. I believe we should focus our time on getting on with living and live each day as if it were our last. We can do the things we know we want in all the major areas of life – spiritually, physically, emotionally, and mentally. We can have more fun and enjoy each day in our work and relationships, both social and intimate and live every day in a body in which we can feel proud. Follow the advice on time in my book and you will always live each day at your optimum level.

Living and thriving in our stressful Twenty-first century lifestyles is not easy. We are bombarded with mixed messages from advertising about living the good life. Too often so many of us are striving and working hard with high levels of stress just to maintain this ideal lifestyle. But how much of the Banana Republic-Lexus-Rolex-Crate & Barrel-house-at-the-beach, high-speed, computer-generated-AOL existence is robbing us of an actual LIFE? If you're stressed to capacity because you need to spend more to support a lifestyle to meet others' expectations, maybe it's time to slow down and ask, "Is sacrificing my day-to-day life worth the cost of maintaining this type of lifestyle? What would I really like to do? How can I slow down, adjust, change or do something new and different? The high-stress lifestyle is harmful to many men. Scientists have proven that enhanced stress leads to lowered testosterone and a higher incidence of heart attacks, strokes, and cancer. We need to slow down and give our bodies a break. Exercise and good eating are two of the best preventative measures to keep physical problems. I aim to arm you for success at a minimum during our prime years.

My experience as a fitness trainer of mature men over forty has given me a special insight into the workings of the human mind and the bodily changes that manifest as we age. One major change is that some men start to feel complacent in an unfit body. Some develop an attitude and state, "Well, why bother to go to the trouble of working out and depriving myself? I'm too old to change."

I've heard this scenario over the years with hundreds of men that have all but given up on hope for changing or creating a better life. The more adventurous men grab life by the neck and swing it around. I admire those who have decided that age means nothing while pursuing a worthwhile fitness goal, whether it's cosmetic (losing 10 pounds) or a sports achievement (running a marathon, competing in a long cross-country bike tour, or even an over-40 basketball league).

The rocking chair scenario of our grandfathers' era when men were expected to stop work at sixty-five and sit in leisure all day is no longer relevant today. In fact, being sedentary and purposeless in retirement is one of the known factors causing premature death of men over seventy. The days of sitting around and dwelling on the past just won't cut it for this new generation who demand an ever-increasing level of sports, fitness, and adventure as they retire and move well into the advanced years.

The definition of retirement has changed as well. We now know that men are more productive and capable in their seventies and beyond than ever before. Exercise and diet play a crucial role in the quality and ultimately the quantity of life. So why not invest in the future and prioritize time for fitness today? Like any good investment, the future dividends will help to create a higher quality lifestyle for you to have fun with and enjoy for years to come.

I want to help you to realize your physical fitness goals, to share my experiences, and to tell the stories of other men who have struggled but ultimately triumphed to a happy end. By sharing the knowledge and specialized insight I have gleaned from my twenty-two years in the fitness business, I hope that you will be inspired to take up your own journey to leading a healthier, happier, and ultimately more fun-filled lifestyle. I advise my clients as they begin this journey to realize that they will have to take small steps at first (baby steps) and gradually build to where they are comfortably challenged on a day-to-day basis. It's not easy, but as you go along you can see dramatic results. You can begin to see changes in your pant size and the mirror can become less intimidating. When you take small steps and succeed, the motivation magnetizes you to continue moving ahead. Your desire to maintain and improve fitness will feel irresistible. My techniques and advice will give you the desired effects if you follow them carefully and consistently. ***<u>Now, get to work and enjoy the journey!</u>***

TIP #2: It's okay to take shortcuts in reaching your fitness goals:

Quality shortcuts can provide the most direct route to truly outstanding fitness success and a feeling of accomplishment. Shortcuts will make your life better if you give them a fair try. I know that traditionally, taking the quickie route is often seen as less of an accomplishment. Many equate longer, more arduous workouts as the most noble and worthy path. ***Right?*** Try again! Teeth gritting, white-knuckled will power and suffering through deprivation *never* works in the long run. No one likes to be in a place of pain or discomfort for too long. I advocate taking the unusual route of lesser resistance and doing what feels right for you within your comfort levels. My strategy will provide greater, long-lasting success. If you want to become your best, consider some of my shortcuts, lighten up your frustration load, and watch what happens.

> "There is no obstacle, no problem, and no difficulty that will keep me from reaching my goal today. I do whatever it takes and I make it happen regardless of circumstances or impossibilities."
> - *Hyrum Smith, creator of Franklin Day Planner*

Most Americans have been spoon-fed thirty to sixty minute solutions to their lifetime problems based on the unreal world of TV and docudramas. We are often impatient when things don't occur at our desired pace. Also, we are longing to make the changes with bodies but we are unable to believe or comprehend the amount of time and daily commitment required to make it a reality. Immediate gratification is all around us in everything we see and do. High-speed Internet, faster cars, mega-fast trains, and instant oatmeal are all examples of modern day human impatience. However, the human body still lives as if it's in the Stone Age. The body hasn't evolved nor caught up with the newer technologies and foods that we eat. That's why so many of us have problems with eating and exercise goals. Because of the snail's pace progress that seems to take too much time with slow, incremental return, shortcuts are more important than ever. I've designed shortcuts to fit into your crazy, tech-driven world while providing the slow steady progress your body needs to make longer-lasting physiological changes. Trust me, it works.

Simplify your life was the mantra during the 1990s, but how realistic is going back to the farm, growing your own food, and getting into horse manure when you have a mortgage, a car payment, and a MasterCard balance. Perhaps the new phrase should be *SHORTCUT YOUR LIFE*. Do it all, but do it in <u>small, tiny bites</u>. Do all the things you feel you need to do in smaller increments. Think of life as a huge restaurant buffet.

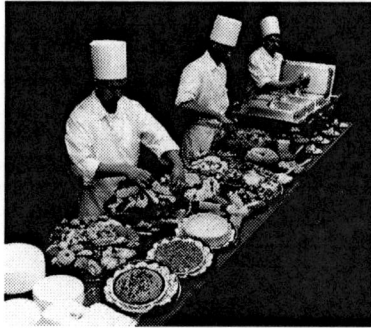

You're at dinner and you want to eat everything (*especially* the dessert), but you know your stomach can only handle so much. So, how can you enjoy it? Take small portions and sample bites so you can control the amount of calories and levels of fullness. Does this sound more appealing than deprivation and missing out?

I use this metaphor when talking to clients about exercise. Just do small amounts consistently. Don't try to bite off more than you can chew too fast. Please, don't be too gung ho for two months and then burnout like a shooting star. Start small and build on each tiny success. The best way to achieve consistency with exercise is to begin and maintain with the shortcut techniques I discuss with you later in this book.

TIP #3: Prioritize fitness as if fitness were a matter of life & death.

I recommend that you try to act as if you are the heart attack survivor who needed to exercise and eat right just to stay alive. During my years as a trainer, the number one excuse I've heard regarding failed fitness attempts is lack of time. The overworked, career-driven American guy gets too busy and easily distracted with a myriad of demands and obligations in his life. So when push comes to shove, the fitness program is often the first thing to go. "Priorities" is what they say. Or, they have one of a myriad of explanations:

"I gotta work."
"I need to devote all my energy to my career."
"It's my family/relationships that get in the way."
"I'm too busy with another hobby/activity."
"I just can't fit one more thing on my schedule!"

The real problem is a lack of motivation along with the fear that achieving fitness goals may not be accomplished. Know this – I can promise you that changes can and do happen. You really can get fit! The single, biggest obstacle to consistently sticking to a program is a lack of prioritizing. Many post-cardio rehab patients and survivors of serious illness are some of the most dedicated fitness enthusiasts. Why? Getting fit and eating nutritional meals had become a matter of life and death. Now there's motivation to prioritize fitness whenever and wherever possible NO MATTER WHAT! But, why wait to feel forced into a corner to get fit and live a healthier lifestyle. If only we could all develop the immediate, do-or-die attitude of the recovering heart surgery patient who must exercise to regain strength to stay alive and healthy.

I believe that there is a distinction to draw between shortcuts and taking the easy way out. Many of my clients have been victims of infomercial scams like the Electronic Ab Machine. Or, some people tried taking huge doses of "fat burners" (herbal speed, ephedrine, and caffeine); others thought the answer was found through taking steroids. Although these products may work temporarily, to attain fitness success still requires a commitment to exercise and diet. Furthermore, pills simply do not magically transform your body overnight. There are many unsafe, unproven methods, scams, diets, machines, and gurus who are preaching an instant magic solution to your diet and exercise problems. Don't believe any of so-called easy, no-hassle claims. They are designed to do one thing – make money for entrepreneurs as a get rich technique. So, buyers beware!

Modern conveniences such as cars, appliances, and computers have made our life better. On the other hand, these conveniences may also make us fat. Modern life has been punctuated by a desire to do less work and enjoy more leisure. However, the truth is and studies show that Americans have been steadily increasing our average workweek since 1977 (***Source***: *United States Department of Commerce*). If more Americans want to enjoy leisure, why then, are 55% of Americans overweight? And, how is it that we rank dead last in the amount of vacation and days off compared to other industrialized countries like Germany, France, and England? We are a nation of strivers and progress is our mantra but our lifestyles are wreaking havoc on the health of our nation.

Here's the scoop: According to a 2001 Gallup poll, only 10% of adults exercise with regularity, and at any given time 75% of us are on some type of diet. Some chuckle, but at least the $10+ billion dollar per year diet industry is still growing and seems recession-proof. The one technology that hasn't yet been developed is one that keeps our bodies in shape while we tend to our modern conveniences, spend our time in cars, and face computer screens all day while eating high-calorie convenience foods. The best technology to date is simply good eating habits and consistent exercise. The techniques here will revolutionize the way you eat, exercise, and manage your whole life.

The ideas I advocate are the result of my twenty-two years in the fitness and nutrition industry, along with the collaboration with and research from some of the best minds in the fields of fitness, psychology, sports, nutrition, and coaching. I encourage you to explore and discover workable solutions to your fitness challenges. The most difficult and arduous task ahead of you is to just get started. The first step is the hardest, but it is the most important. Congratulate yourself! Just by reading this text, you have made a start and are head and shoulders above the other 90% of the population whom are still just talking about starting an exercise routine and making a new life.

Recent innovations in the fitness field have made shortcuts the way to reach your optimum levels. Engineered foods, life-enhancing supplements, and vitamins are part of our daily diet and cut some corners. Here's a short list of machines that assist my clients with shortcuts:

- Treadmill
- EFX Elliptical Trainer
- Computerized heart rate monitor
- Portable VO2 analyzers.

The science of longevity has become a new field in medicine. We have discovered drugs that circumvent the aging process. Doctors across the country are opening up "anti-aging clinics" and "longevity centers" to promote healthy lifestyles and better living. Through the use of prescriptions such as growth hormone testosterone, estrogen, and a regimen of natural herbs that work synergistically with a healthy diet and exercise program, doctors seek to help men live and look more youthful into their advanced years. Physical therapists and rehab specialists are using artificial body parts to replace limbs, organs, and stem cell research promises a whole new world of disease-free living. Keep in mind that the new frontiers of medicine are cutting limits from aging, improving our health and overall well-being *(**Ask your doctor for more information)*.

Pain relief for arthritis and other autoimmune disorders associated with aging and joint degradation has advanced light years ahead of aspirin and other old fashioned remedies. Further, there are very few diseases today that we cannot in some way either control or arrest progression. Until the mid-1990s, an AIDS or HIV diagnosis was akin to an early death sentence. Until recently, most cancers were deadly and uncontrollable and living an active lifestyle into your nineties was nothing more than a pipe dream. I have a client whose grandfather still caddied two golf bags at a time through his mid-eighties and competed in the Senior Olympics as a long-distance runner at age 87 (client Perry Monastero's grandfather Sam Monastero of Norristown, Pennsylvania)! The same client's grandmother had a double mastectomy in 1975 and almost 30 years later is still running around, driving, and traveling 3 months per year at 88. With our lives so busy and active doesn't it make sense to live life to the fullest in a fully-functioning body that is unrestricted or unencumbered by handicaps, disease, restrictions, lack of functional ability or low energy? Investing even a minimal amount of time into some form of physical activity has been shown to increase the quality and quantity of life. In 2001, the American College of Sports Medicine (ACSM, January 2002) released its recommended quota for the health benefits of exercise and it was surprising, especially to those of us in the fitness business. ACSM studied the healthiest adults and found that they engaged in a minimum of only 20 minutes per day of moderate activity. Activities such as gardening, housework, walking to work, raking leaves, scrubbing floors, and chopping wood are ideal for improving one's health and spirit. Researchers found that compared to zero exercise, a mere three, ten-minute sessions spread over the course of a day could create a positive effect! Talk about shortcuts to fitness!

So you *can* squeeze in the minimum with almost no effort at all. Keep in mind that these studies were done to show the *minimum* amount required for good overall cardiovascular health and disease prevention. This type of regimen will not give you bulging biceps or washboard abs, but it might encourage more exercise-TV-watching-couch-potatoes to just **do** something! Start now!

Improving the Quality and Quantity of Life

Face it, you *are* going to get older and if things keep advancing we'll all be living to an average of 100 years. It's so important to enjoy your life and feel good in the body you've been given to carry you through this journey. We all want to sample from the big buffet of living. I think the best way to enjoy our long life is to live healthy and make wise choices.

Life's activities and choices are endless. I know that if you are like most, you will want to do it all to enjoy all of life's pleasures while simultaneously and gracefully deal with the pain associated with aging. It might not surprise you to find that the best prescription to make it all happen is exercise. Exercise is the youth elixir (and it's much cheaper than growth hormone treatments) since it keeps us feeling sharp mentally, physically, emotionally, and sexually. As humans, our natural instinct is to feel drawn toward pleasure and away from pain. Exercise if often viewed as an uncomfortable, unpleasant activity. I say this for one simple reason: if gratification from exercise felt as immediate and good as sex or eating, the gyms of America would be filled to capacity.

Jim Hart, A.C.E.

How do you find the enjoyment in exercise? The key when starting out or renewing your commitment is to begin with small doses. Use the shortcuts I will mention and be mindful that the first 15 minutes of any exercise activity might bring howls of protest from your body. It is natural for the body to want to remain as it is. This tendency is called "homeostasis." We also call it inertia. Once you get over the threshold of 15 minutes, your body finally gets the idea and will make all the necessary physiological adjustments to make you more comfortable and your body soon adapts to this heightened state of activity. Remember, exercise is an intrusion on your body at first, but the pleasure will come as the brain sends out signals to release the feel-good chemicals (also called endorphins). Once you overcome that hurdle, you will begin to feel better. Have a little patience and wait for your body to feel energized. It's often smooth sailing from then on.

The small steps you take can pay off with tremendous results. As you begin to tap into fat reserves for energy, you build your cardiovascular system, strengthen your heart, increase lung capacity, building both muscle stamina and energy stores. The real payoff comes later when your metabolism stays elevated for up to 12 hours (depending on activity and intensity) and your body burns more calories even while resting!. Exercising is like putting money in the bank; your sweat reaps big dividends soon after and compounds them with interest even after you're done. Taking even the smallest steps each day such as simply twenty minutes of walking or taking the stairs will provide you significant rewards in fat loss and better health.

The shortcuts to fitness in the chapters that follow provide you with quick solutions and pathways that will lead to your ultimate success on your fitness journey. You can take pride in your efforts however minor they seem – in the end, they will all add up. These small building blocks slowly come together to help you build a rock-solid foundation of health, wellness and a muscular, low-fat body that will serve you well into the Twenty-first century!

Tip #4: Find Time to Exercise

If I had to make my list of top ten problems people have with starting a fitness program, again I'd say that finding time to exercise would be at the top. The problem starts when one starts looking to find some spare time to fit in exercise. The concept of spare time is a fallacy. No one has spare time. Time is like spare money – you can choose to budget or spend it any way you like, but none of it is extra, none of it is ever "spare."

Time is the great equalizer. Both the poorest and the wealthiest people on Earth all possess the same 24 hours. So, forget about finding extra time in your already overbooked schedule. Let's find ways to budget the time and create the life you love that includes fitting in all the activities that you value and the things you want to do – especially with your body.

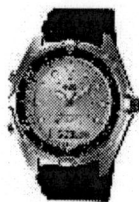

As a personal example: in the writing of this book, it took a tremendous initial effort to budget my time. I always found excuses and better or more urgent things to do. Anything *aside* from WRITING. Writers are procrastinators. It's easy to find ways to avoid the computer when you just don't feel like it or have too many other responsibilities. But, successful writers (like successful exercisers) don't have any more minutes in the day than unsuccessful writers. Some of the most successful writers of today worked full-time jobs and carried out the duties of parenting while writing before anyone ever heard of them. J.K. Rowling, author of the <u>Harry Potter</u> book series was a destitute single mother who wrote longhand in coffee shops while her baby napped beside her. John Grisham worked 60-hour weeks as a lawyer and rose at the crack of dawn each day before his wife and kids awoke to write <u>A Time to Kill</u>. It took him three years to complete. For me, these two authors serve as role models and inspiration.

"Finding the time" is a myth that keeps you stuck in your same way of thinking, and being. The problem is not time, it's **HABIT DEVELOPMENT**. **IT'S TAKING SOMETHING THAT YOU'RE NOT USED TO DOING AND TURNING IT INTO SOMETHING YOU CANNOT DO WITHOUT.** Work on this plan for habit acquisition and the time deficits will take care of itself.

So, how do you build a new, positive habit? I give you the example of teaching the game of catch with a little kid who can barely get his hands around the ball and is just learning to throw. What do you do? Do you throw the ball as hard and fast as you can toward the child? Of course not! It would be impossible for him to catch it and he would get completely frustrated and give up. Watch an experienced father teaching his kid to play baseball. How does he pitch those first balls? Easy and gently, slow and underhand. So, why is it done like that? Because he wants the child to develop his skill and he wants the kid to feel like a winner. Skill-building starts slowly, a little at a time. When the kid gets good at catching the ball with an easy throw and good at hitting the ball from an easy pitch, then the father pitches marginally harder. He keeps the challenge level slightly above the child's skill level so the kid's abilities can grow step-by-step. Therefore, the son's efforts are reinforced with a feeling of success.

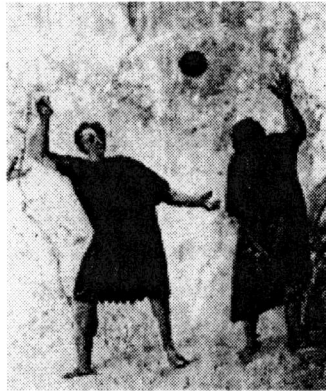

At the risk of being obvious why is it done this way? <u>Because no one likes to be lousy at doing something</u>. If you keep having an unsuccessful experience with something you stop doing it. It's not fun to fail.

And failing from over-estimating initial goals is what most people have done with their exercise programs. Most people bite off a too big chunk right at the beginning and find they can't chew it, so they spit it out and stop completely and then blame it on "NOT HAVING ENOUGH TIME." If you are going to teach yourself something new whether it's playing ball, speaking French, or learning to cook, think of yourself as that small child trying to catch a ball. If you start with a ridiculous goal like "I'm going to run an hour every day, five days a week," it would be like throwing a curving fastball to a six-year-old who never played catch before. You will quickly feel frustrated and ultimately give up.

So, how do you make it happen? How do you stack the deck in your favor for long-term success? You have to set up the game so you can win! You must learn to use the power of the subconscious mind. Your subconscious mind is very simplistic and very digital. It knows two states: ON & OFF, SUCCESS & FAILURE. If you set yourself up an initial goal like thirty minutes on the treadmill and you only do 26 minutes, whether you are aware of it or not, your subconscious logs that as a failure. You aimed for 30 and you didn't make it, you say to yourself. Somewhere in your subconscious mind is a little gremlin sticking its tiny tongue out and yelling, "LOSER!" But, if you set a goal of five minutes and you do five minutes, your mind logs that _as a win_.

Does it matter that it's only five minutes? Not at all! What matters when you start out is that you had a positive experience.

In the first months of exercise, all I want you to try to do is log a set of positives. In the beginning, we're in the habit-building mode, not in the "How much exercise did I do?" mode. It is not important **HOW MUCH YOU DO. WHAT IS IMPORTANT IS THAT YOU DO <u>SOMETHING</u>** and <u>do it consistently</u>. That's how we build a habit successfully.

I start all my new clients on a simple walking program ten minutes at a time, three times per week. This consistency helps to log in those little victories in the subconscious and gradually build a habit. This registers in your mind that exercise (no matter how long or intense) is always a **WIN** situation for you!

You might be skeptical and say, "Ten minutes can't possibly make a difference." But you're dead wrong. It does make a difference because more important than anything is the fact that <u>you've kept your promise to yourself</u>. You said you would do ten minutes a day, three times per week and you did exactly that! You've kept your word to yourself which is the most important lesson in habit development. You are learning to believe that when you say something, it happens. This is the secret weapon of habit development and time management.

I once trained a man named Dennis who was fifty pounds overweight. He had never exercised successfully, hated the discomfort from exercise, and didn't see how he could possibly fit training into his busy schedule. But, he reluctantly came to the gym and tried weights and aerobics. He gave exercise a chance. Soon, he found them dull and tedious and eventually gave up, abandoning his routine within a few weeks. Dennis hired me as a last ditch effort on a friend's recommendation. Our first session was just talking about goals and lifestyle so that I could learn more about Dennis's needs and challenges. The next session, we walked side by side on the treadmill – for only three minutes. Yes, just three minutes! That was his assignment for the next two weeks. Three minutes on the treadmill every other day. When he completed this, he upped the time to four minutes. Can you see how we were conditioning his subconscious here? Small, successful baby steps done with consistency create a favorable environment for developing and maintaining a habit.

The biggest mistake people make when it comes to incorporating exercise into their lives is concentrating on the **amount** they do and how quickly it will produce results. That's the wrong focus. Until it becomes something you can't imagine living without, the focus should be simply on doing something consistently. If you started with as little as one minute a day and over the next two months added no more than 30 seconds a day, you'd be up to a half-hour of exercise.

You can always up the ante once you develop the habit. The real trick is developing the habit. Incidentally, Dennis became one of my most successful clients. He lost weight (sixty pounds!), runs marathons, and lifts weights at our gym five times a week. He looks and feels better than ever.

You can do it too! If exercise is new to you (or you are starting over for roughly the 20th time), treat the initial first weeks of your program as a test of keeping your word. It doesn't matter how little you do. What matters is that you promise to do it and then keep that promise to yourself.

Tip #5: Remember the Pyramid – Food First, Strength Second, Aerobics Third

By focusing on food as a top priority, I am emphasizing just how incredibly important healthy, nutritious eating is. No matter how much you run, no matter how much you lift weights or walk to work, it is useless unless you're eating correctly. Most men are under the impression they can balance out a poor diet by running an extra 15 minutes or going higher on their bench press – they're dead wrong. You can never spend enough time and energy to compensate for a pizza and cheesesteak diet. It takes an hour of running a 9-minute mile for a 160-pound man to burn off a cheeseburger and french-fries. Or, two hours of walking, or 90 minutes on the elliptical trainer. Who has that kind of time? <u>Most of us have a life outside the gym.</u>

Eating Right is the #1 Way to Be Successful in Getting the Body You Want

Eating the right foods is the single most important factor in a successful body makeover program. If you did nothing else (without strength training or aerobic work) you would still see a significant body change by selecting the right foods.

Myth: If I workout more, I won't have to adjust my eating habits to lose weight.

Exercise can create a calorie deficit but it's inefficient to do so without regulating your food intake. Why not just eat a little less and do your regular ½ hour to 40 minutes and create a nice moderate calorie deficit that will gradually add up to a steady fat loss? You can do that without all the teeth-gritting strain and pain of marathon-length workouts.

Think of your program as a pyramid. The base that supports it is the eating (the most important), the middle is the strength training with its muscle building and metabolism-boosting effects, and, finally at the top and the third is cardiovascular training and exercise. Its most important function is to create a healthy heart, a strong set of lungs, and clear clean arteries that are free of cholesterol plaque. A good side effect is the calories burned and the additional fat burned in the process.

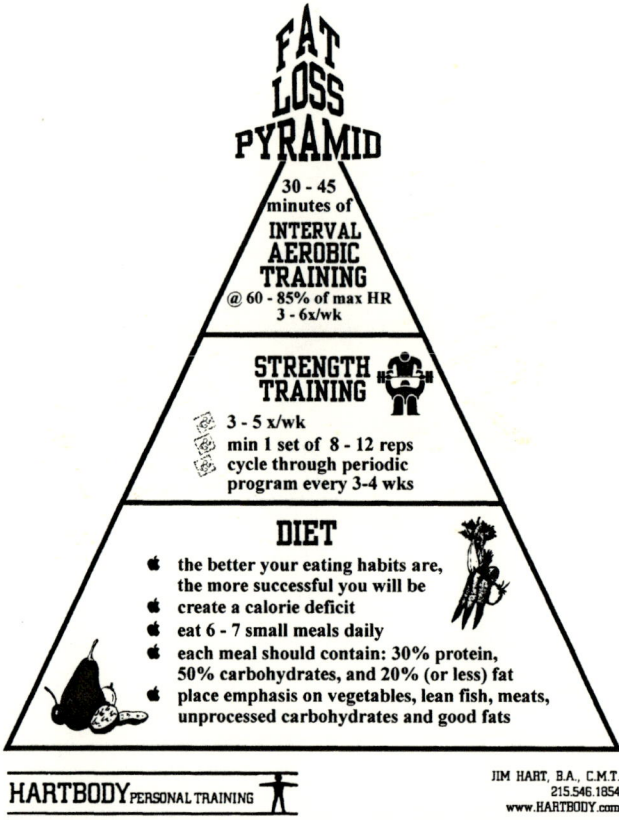

FAT LOSS PYRAMID

30 - 45 minutes of INTERVAL AEROBIC TRAINING
@ 60 - 85% of max HR
3 - 6x/wk

STRENGTH TRAINING
3 - 5 x/wk
min 1 set of 8 - 12 reps
cycle through periodic program every 3-4 wks

DIET
- the better your eating habits are, the more successful you will be
- create a calorie deficit
- eat 6 - 7 small meals daily
- each meal should contain: 30% protein, 50% carbohydrates, and 20% (or less) fat
- place emphasis on vegetables, lean fish, meats, unprocessed carbohydrates and good fats

HARTBODY PERSONAL TRAINING

JIM HART, B.A., C.M.T.
215.546.1854
www.HARTBODY.com

The last word on what is most important is to eat right and support all your efforts towards the body you want. It's not easy but it works and you won't be happy with your body until you make it a habit. So what is the best eating plan for you? Eating is an individual and very personal issue that involves numerous factors such as job, cooking skills, taste, time management, moods, convenience, social/cultural/family upbringing, and goals for body aesthetic and overall health.

Tip #6: Know Your Calorie Needs & Keep a Journal

A complicated and tough area for many trainers is to try to advise our clients on the way to eat for fat loss. If it were so easy to just follow a few rules then why do so many fail? Some personal trainers really believe there is a cookie-cutter, one-size-fits-all diet plan for all of their clients. It's just not true.

Designing an eating plan is a highly individualized undertaking and the sooner you recognize this, the more successful you will be. Simply put, the diet that works best is the one that fits into your lifestyle and fills your needs. Let's try to make this complex issue as simple as possible. Sometimes the easiest and most straightforward plan is the one that you'll stick with, especially if you feel comfortable with it. I use the acronym **K.I.S.S.E.D**: **Keep It Super-Simple Every Day**. Keep the rules and the choices to a minimum. Find a selection of 15 - 20 different foods you really enjoy (*Hey, this doesn't include daily helpings of pepperoni pizza and cheesecake!*) and stay with them.

Be lazy if you have to. Use frozen Lean Cuisine™ meals, canned soup, tuna fish, instant oatmeal, or store-bought rotisserie chicken as part of your eating regimen. Occasionally, go off your plan if you want and try something new, but for the majority of the time do the same thing and you will not have to think or worry about it too much. So, how much of all those simple good foods do you need? In other words, within what calorie range should you be to feel good while losing fat and gaining muscle at the same time?

Tip #7: Caveman Diet

The simplest and easiest weight loss plan ever devised is called the ***Caveman Eating Plan***. You eat everything in its most natural and unprocessed state. Our ancestors, the Caveman, had no flour, sugar, oil, alcohol, or processed meats. They ate a diet mostly vegetarian-based, with lots of fruits, vegetables, greens, nuts, and seeds. They occasionally killed wild animals and caught fish, birds, and whatever was available.

Now, I do not expect you to implement a diet as stringent as a caveman. We will never live up to that style of eating in Twenty-first century America, but by striving to follow this 80% of the time, you will notice dramatic results in the shortest time possible.

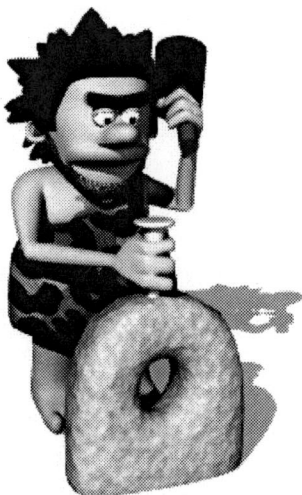

The clients who are most able to strictly follow this plan are amazed at how quickly it changes their body composition. Why not do a little experiment yourself and try it just for five days and see for yourself? You might just feel more energetic and also feel a change in your waistline. Just eliminate flour, sugar, alcohol, and processed meats from your eating Monday through Friday (then splurge if you need it on the weekend). Eat as many vegetables, lean protein (choose lean protein like egg whites, chicken breast, and fish), and greens as you want (<u>don't even count the calories</u>). Eat fruit for dessert and go easy on the potatoes and starches such as rice and pasta. You will give your body a jump-start and start looking leaner and sooner! **Think Big!**

Sample Menus: A Day in the Life of a Caveman

Here's a typical day of food choices, compromises, and real world eating for a Caveman living in the Twenty-first century. This menu is just one sample from a client's diet journal:

Breakfast
> 7:00 a.m. 12 oz cottage cheese, one apple, coffee

Snack
> 9:45 a.m. Pure Protein™ bar (Choose a lower carb bar [5-15g] w/high protein,
> [20 -35g], and low to moderate fat [4-8g].)

Lunch
> 12:00 p.m. (on the run) Subway turkey sandwich (under 300 calories) w/o cheese, double the meat, lettuce, tomatoes, mustard, and pickles and no-fat TCBY™ yogurt for dessert
>
> 2:30 p.m. Granny Smith apple

Snack
> 4:30 p.m. Balance Gold Bar™

Dinner
> 7:00 p.m. Dinner at restaurant—appetizer: mixed green salad (dressing on side) and the entrée: grilled salmon (no sauce), double serving of steamed broccoli (asked server to hold the rice), split half of the dessert (splurge)

Snack
> 10:00 p.m. 2 light yogurts and a ¼ cup of blueberries

Tip #8: Volumize!

Another way to lose weight quickly is a technique called **Volumizing**. How does volumizing work? Most of your food choices are selected from the "wet carbs" family. Wet carbs include green and other colorful vegetables, fibrous leafy salad greens, fruit and highly unprocessed grains such as oats, brown rice, wheat germ, and barley. These foods add bulk to your diet without adding high amounts of calories. They let you eat more food without storing fat. It works like magic.

Tip #9: Fiberize!

The bonus is the additional fiber you'll add keeps your internal plumbing healthy and promotes anti-cancer fighting properties in the large intestine. **For each gram of fiber you add, you subtract one gram of carbohydrate.** For men trying to be careful with their carb intake for weight loss reasons, this is great news. For example, a 4-ounce serving of broccoli contains 20 grams of carbs and 7 grams of fiber. That means you are only getting 13 grams of carbohydrates. The fiber passes the food through and the cellulose in the food is indigestible and acts like a Roto-Rooter scrub brush.

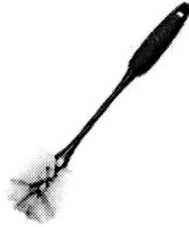

Eat more, weigh less by looking for ways to get extra fruit, vegetables, and whole grains in your diet. Some ideas:
- Double-up on the veggies and eat only half the starch rice or white potatoes;
- Add Fiber One™ or All Bran Extra Fiber™ to your oatmeal or eat it raw with milk or sprinkled on yogurt or cottage cheese; and,
- Add sliced vegetables to scrambled eggs, and serve with multi-grain bread.

According to the American Dietetic Association spokeswoman Connie Diekman, fiber-full foods are nature's appetite suppressant. Another good reason to fiberize: The U.S. Department of Agriculture found in a 1997 study that for each gram of fiber in your meal, your body subtracts seven calories. The Harvard Medical School discovered that fiber can lower cholesterol levels. Plus, why not eat more fiber when foods inherently found with fiber are usually tasty and lower in fat than most other things found

Jim Hart, A.C.E.

in most American diets? Additionally, fiber-rich foods naturally contain greater portions of vitamins and minerals. There are numerous other special findings that I want to share. Keep in mind that fiberizing truly works. This strategy injects more energy and holds cravings under control, keeping you healthier overall.

Tip #10: Know the Always/Sometimes/Never Food List

To be truly successful you will need to be conscious of making food choices that support your goals of a healthy, low-fat body. Always ask yourself, "Is this supporting my cause? Is this food helping me to realize my body potential? Will something else satisfy me, or can I just eat a small portion?" Keep this abbreviated list handy and use it as a guide.

Remember that there are no forbidden foods – only forbidden ways of eating them. We all have our "Trigger Foods." What is it about trigger foods that I feel is important to know? Well, for some people a trigger food is Haagen-Dazs® ice cream. For others, it's a fast-food double cheeseburger. Identify for yourself what your trigger foods are and be mindful of when you are feeling the pang for something your body craves. You can learn to lose your cravings, but you need to remember that _**you**_ have control. If a cookie has been calling you all day, try eating half and give the rest to a kid or feed the birds with the leftover portion. Don't feel guilty about waste. I always say, *"If you eat the waste it goes to your waist!"* Start looking at the foods you love as items you can still have, but consume **LESS** or **SMALLER** portions of those trigger foods.

We all know the "red light" foods. These "forbidden foods" include anything with extra sugar, butter, cream, and yes I'm going to mention anything deep-fried. Here is a partial list of foods categorized by their value in <u>my quick fat loss and low fat maintenance program</u>:

Jim Hart, A.C.E.

Red Light	Yellow Light	Green Light
STOP & THINK	*PROCEED w/CAUTION*	*GO!!*
Occasional Treats	**Moderate Amounts**	**As Much As You Want**
anything dipped in chocolate	Lean beef	green vegetables
fast foods	Lean chicken	radishes, onions
honey nuts	Fish, eggs, skim milk	mushrooms, celery
frozen ice cream	Fat-free dairy, cheese	fat-free dressings
most sweet cold cereals	fat-free yogurt	egg whites
big thick fat steaks	whole grain bread	water chestnuts
prime rib	low fat crackers, chips	diet soda, Krystal Lite™
lamb chops	frozen yogurt	fat free soups
lunch meat	lite processed cheese	zucchini, cucumbers
Philadelphia steak sandwich	light cheese pizza	blueberries, raspberries
Pretzels	sweet potatoes	water, diet tonic water
Hoagies	fat free ice cream	wheat germ
Tastycakes™	oranges, bananas	melons

Tip #11: Eliminate all or nothing thinking

The 80/20 rule is a good way to eat. The previously mentioned 'Caveman' diet is a good representation of a real life eating style that's altogether neither perfect nor totally free of sugar, flour, and fats. The typical calendar day shows that our model client kept to it 80% of the time and that's what counts. At the end of each week, this client usually earned a calorie deficit to maintain a steady weight loss of 1-2 pounds per week. Make good to excellent choices roughly 80% of the time and you'll still come out ahead. This eliminates that "***ALL OR NOTHING THINKING***" that leads to going off your diet and bingeing.

Tip #12: Avoid fad diets and explore good diets

I believe that you will want to avoid certain diets that are extremely difficult to maintain. Your psyche just doesn't want to live with a stringent, over-disciplined manner of eating. <u>There are several diets I recommend that you should avoid if you want a long-term result for your efforts</u>. The following all-or-nothing diets have exacerbated my clients and millions like them:

- Dr. Atkins (or any severe carb-restricted diet)
- Jenny Craig (or pre-packaged meal plans)
- LA Weight Loss (or *any* plan that uses herbal stimulants and appetite suppressants)
- Protein Power (or any diet that severely limits or restricts one type of food or emphasizes too much of one food group over another)

Okay, it's true. Several popular American diets, such as the ones listed above work for short-term weight loss and many individuals rave about them. According to Dr. Kelly Brownell, an eating disorder specialist at Harvard, most (about 95%) people will return to their original weight or a ***higher*** weight within 6 to 24 months. Taking a moderate approach in a slower and more manageable way doesn't sound as dramatic or exciting as the promises of these quick weight-loss solutions but the results over the long-term are more permanent and lasting.

Besides my own series of plans, I think there are many sound weight loss programs that will help you to take weight off without driving you crazy with rules and restrictions and relapses and weight gain.

Here are a few programs that my clients and I have found helpful:

- E-Diet.com (I find this website to have the best information and diet support)
- Dietstogo.com (A healthy food home delivery service for busy people)
- Weight Watchers

- **T.O.P.S.** or, **T**ake **O**ff **P**ounds **S**ensibly (This hospital-based program can be found by checking your local hospital's dietary department for ongoing programs for sensible weight loss)
- The Pritkin Plan
- American Heart Association diet books and programs from Dr. Dean Ornish
- Cliff Sheats *Lean Bodies* series
- Dr. Shapiro's "*Picture Perfect Weight Loss*" program
- The Volumetrics Diet
- *Prevention Magazine*'s "Get Thin, Get Young"
- Body for Life, by Bill Phillips (a structured body-building program)

Tip #13: Hire experts to help

Another strategy that works: hire a registered dietician to tap into the knowledge and skills of a professional (see Web Resources). There are many great weight-loss and support group programs sponsored by local hospitals. Check your areas and local phone directory for availability. All of these offer simple long-term and realistic plans for losing weight and living a healthier lifestyle. Find a registered dietitian online at American Dietetic Association's National Nutrition Network (http://www.eatright.org/find.html.). Or, visit Pounds Aweigh (http://www.poundsaweigh.com). For those clients facing the stress of an eating disorder, I might recommend Rader Programs (http://www.raderprograms.com) or Eating Disorder Counseling, (http://www.eatingdisordercounseling.com) Inc.

Tip #14: Eat six times a day and lose fat faster

Keeping your blood sugar steady throughout the day is the key to managing hunger and keeping off weight. The idea of grazing on small meals or snacks (*we call it practicing "SAFE SNAX"*) helps to keep your metabolism running at a higher rate. You can eliminate tough and dangerous cravings and avoid dips in energy by stabilizing your blood sugar. As a result, you will feel more alive and satisfied with extra zing. The body is like a furnace: the more fuel you give it, the hotter it will run. If you're burning hotter and higher, you're also burning more fat calories, too. Eat six times a day to greatly reduce hunger pangs, keep blood sugar levels moderate, and your fat burning metabolism full speed ahead.

Tip #15: Learn the value of a cheat day

Having a food splurge once in a while is a fantastic way to balance your healthy eating and your cravings for junk food. You don't have to give up your favorite foods altogether on the **Personal Trainer Secrets** program. I realize it's not easy giving up the foods you like even 80% of the time and most people are worn down in their resolve to stay "clean" after 2-3 weeks of strict will-power enforced healthy eating. The Cheat Day is a safety valve that allows a build-up to release before an explosion (or binge) can occur. For example, one of my clients can walk by Dunkin' Donuts® only for so many times without eventually giving in. So, have fun with your Cheat Day — make a whole day out of it (some people like to make it Sunday; others choose to spread out their splurges over a week (i.e., when they are going to a special restaurant or celebrating a special holiday).

A balanced approach will help you maintain your plan for a lifetime. Remember, your body does not gain weight after one meal. You gain the same way you lose, slowly and methodically over a period of days, weeks, and months. So, cheat once or twice a week and do it guilt-free. And cheat with the confidence of knowing you are still going to reach your weight-loss goal.

Tip #16: Eat for long-term health maintenance

I would like you to develop an eating strategy that is actually my own secret to weight control maintenance. Rollercoaster dieting is the worst possible situation for a man who wants a low-fat, muscular body. Going on a strict fad diet followed by going off it and then rushing into a totally undisciplined style of eating makes your body look awful and takes its toll on your psyche. There's more bad news: each time you lose and regain it becomes harder to lose extra pounds. The body will kick and scream and fight to protect giving up its fat stores because it thinks you are going to starve it again!

The satisfaction in taking a long-term, moderate approach comes from the ease of taking a more relaxed, less perfectionist approach that allows for occasional lapses where you might regain a few pounds from a vacation, a stressful life event (death, divorce, job loss, etc.) or a dramatic lifestyle change. Take it in stride and just pick up and keep going. Begin with the next meal if you lapse. **A relapse**, on the other hand, is a total backslide into old habits with a corresponding gain in fat, **a lapse** is only temporary and is just a small blip on the screen. You can recover easily from a short lapse and still maintain your body goals.

When you are trying to reach your optimal calorie range, other important factors to consider are activity level, lowered testosterone, and exercise intensity. As you age, the level of free testosterone gradually declines with each decade, causing increased levels of fat storage and lowered amounts of muscle building. You don't need the same amount of calories at 50 as you did when you were 25. This is not because you are eating more. Rather, it's because testosterone increases muscle mass that increases metabolism. As your testosterone levels decrease, so does your metabolism and your body's need for calories.

Feeling happy with your food plan by setting realistic moderate goals is more important than gritting your teeth and suffering through deprivation and the sober discipline of a restricted diet plan. Pleasure and satisfaction are key elements to staying on an eating program that fits into your daily routine. After all we're hard-wired to move toward pleasure and away from pain.

33

Deep down, every person knows what works for them. I believe that there is no **ONE-SIZE-FITS-ALL APPROACH** when it comes to eating. Beating yourself up, comparing yourself to other people, or blaming your lack of will power is unproductive and bad for your self-esteem. Instead, honor and be proud of your weaknesses, work with them so they have a place in your plan, but do it on your terms and within the boundaries of common sense. If you're a pizza fanatic, have it once or twice a week at a restaurant with friends, or make a date out of it. Don't deny your need for it. The cravings eventually return at some point as a binge and crash. Keep a loose hand on the reins of diet control. Sometimes you will need to pull tight, other times you will loosen up and just coast. The wise way is to take the middle road, be moderate, and above all, be happy.

Tip #17: Increase exercise intensity

Increasing exercise intensity levels can offset the body's natural decrease in testosterone as we age. Also, consider having your testosterone levels checked by your physician to make sure they aren't abnormally low. A few of my clients improved muscle building and fitness while on a doctor-supervised plan of hormone boosting therapy. Ask your doctor—it may well be worth it. In men over 40, a lowering of muscle mass is a precursor to the "middle age spread." You can beat the spread as you age, but the older you get, the more diligent and watchful you must be. Also, as I mentioned earlier, testosterone levels are working against you as are other lifestyle factors including injuries, joint and back restrictions, time demands, as well as the mental blocks of "Why should I care, I'm getting older?" Or, "What do you expect, I'm 52?!"

Numerous university-based studies have shown the key to metabolic fat burning in men is a phenomenon called E.P.O.C., or *exercise, post-oxygen consumption*. Scientists set out to find what kind of exercise produces the highest metabolism boosting oxygen and energy consumption after the workout. Not surprisingly, they found that the more intense the exercise, the better the post-oxygen consumption (*ACSM Review*, **March 1999**). You can achieve amazing results by giving it your all when strength training or going a little faster during your cardio session. Think of the difference between an Olympic sprinter who goes hard and fast for a short period and a marathon runner who goes long and slower. The one is super-muscular and lean, the other is lean, but mostly skin and bones.

From *National Strength and Conditioning Association* editor Paul Roetert: **EPOC** can be compared to the process of getting a charcoal barbecue grill going. You first need to ignite a high flame fueled by lighter fluid. Then, after the roaring fire dies down, the Briquettes™ stay hot, burning steadily for several hours. Your body operates the same way. Give it a quick, short burst of high-intensity. Then when you're done, your muscle cells burn a slow steady source of energy (fat) while repairing and building more muscle.

Being intense during your strength workout has numerous benefits. It increases your release of growth hormone, essential for muscle growth, it releases those feel-good endorphins that give you a mental and emotional boost and it enhances your sex drive by increasing testosterone levels. More muscle, a natural high, and a drug-free aphrodisiac – what more could you ask for? Do your next workout with all-out intensity and eschew distractions to diminish your resolve. The NIKE™ ads are corny but ring true for athletic pursuits. The message: Don't think about it—JUST DO IT!

Tip #18: Build muscle to increase metabolism

We have begun to discuss eating. A close second and very important thing you can do in getting a buff body is strength training on a regular and consistent basis. Building muscle mass is the key to both a better body and to lowering fat levels. An incredible method to look better and fast is to lift weights and maintain a good eating program. One will work without the other, but the combo of both will create a super double-whammy that speeds your progress immensely.

Myth: "Lifting weights makes me bulky."
Metabolically-active muscle tissue is my magic secret to burning additional fat with less effort, without excessive amounts of aerobics, and without tight food restrictions. A higher metabolism means your body draws more from fat stores as its primary source of fuel to keep your energy levels up and to maintain life-sustaining functions like digestion, breathing, heartbeat, brain activity, and cell reproduction. Higher metabolism through muscle mass is like putting your body on a long slow simmer all day long. As the hours, days, and months pass, the body gradually decreases these fat stores (provided you eat reasonably).

Tip #19: Don't overdo cardio

Aerobic exercise is not a magic fat-burning solution to a poor diet. Many people believe aerobics is the answer to losing body fat. Think of aerobics as the opposite of muscle metabolism – a flambé of cherries jubilee, a quick calorie-burning flash that lasts for a limited amount of time that is brief, sustained by the ignition of refined sugar (alcohol). Let your body work for you and burn fat the easy way – lift weights two to three times (or more) per week and enjoy the results. Coupled with aerobic exercise, you'll see results FAST!

Doing Lots of Cardio But Not Losing Weight?

One of the problems is that most of us over-estimate the amount of calories we burn particularly on indoor exercise machines like the Treadmill™, EFX™ (elliptical trainer), and Stair-Stepper™. The calorie counts on those machines incorporate your basal metabolic rate, which measures the calories you burn anyway to fuel your vital functions such as breathing and digestion.

Here's an example: If a 180 lb. man works out on the Stairmaster™ for thirty minutes at level five, he'd burn 230 calories, but only 193 more if he sat at home reading. At that rate, he would need to do 18 Stairclimber™ workouts to lose on pound of fat rather than the 15 workouts the machine readings imply.

Myth: "I do not have the time to fit in working out."

I've addressed time crunches previously, but it deserves a great deal of attention. If you can allot three hours out of a 168-hour week, you will see dramatic results especially if you haven't lifted before. If you consider the small amount of time required for a large and worthwhile return, it makes sense to put it in your schedule. Prioritizing the three hours a week is the key to being consistent. You prioritize taking showers, going to work, movies, religion, and doctor appointments. Why not give strength training the same gravity of importance?

Remember, the rewards are immediate and gratifying as well as long-lasting. You feel an endorphin rush as daily stress can be released with a few sets of bench pressing. Grunting and groaning lets out those primal emotions and just going to a gym where everyone is doing something positive and wonderful for their bodies and minds can remove from your problems for a while. Besides, there's great music, beautiful people, possible dates, all available in a clean, healthy, smoke-free environment.

Again, strength training beats cardiovascular training for men over 40 who need to lose body fat. I can't stress this enough. I'm not saying that aerobic exercise isn't something you should avoid; I think it's vitally important especially for a healthy heart and its disease fighting capabilities. The point is this – if <u>had to choose between strength training or cardio work, I want your choice to be strength training *along with diet work*</u>. In fact, weight training has been shown to reduce cardiac risk factors in men according to a landmark study (*American Medicine Association Journal*, October 2002).

Tip #20: Short workouts are best for men over 40!

Studies show that keeping workouts short and intense makes for a happy and healthier forty-plus year-old. Long, grueling workout routines like the ones in the popular bodybuilding magazines give an unrealistic view of how you should train, even if you are as young as the guys found in the pictures of fitness magazines. The training I advocate is about 45 minutes to 1 hour (maximum). After that, you reach a point of diminishing returns and may actually lower your testosterone levels. Long-term success in training comes from committing a small amount of time daily to exercise. 45 minutes is a more manageable and realistic goal for most men who lead full and busy career, activity, and family-oriented lives.

Furthermore, researchers (*Journal of the American College of Nutrition* 20 (5): 494-501, 2001) have discovered that short sessions of cardio produce similar results when compared to one longer session. Given this finding, why not try combining a few different exercise sessions over a period of the week and do it in small bites? Who wants to do a long, boring aerobic session at the end of a strength training workout. Instead, you could end your workout with something enjoyable. Try going for a quick walk, race walk, run, jog, stair climb, train on the EFX machine, shoot some hoops, throw a Frisbee around, play racquetball, jump rope – the list could go on. I think trying small amounts of cardio that you enjoy most might work out for you, especially as I know that most of my clients lead active lives and don't want to do a long, boring 35-minute aerobic exercise at the end of a strength training workout.

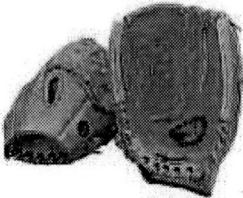

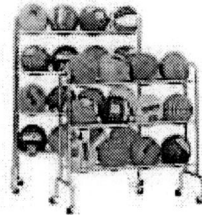

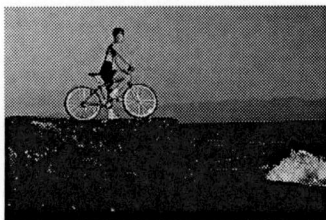

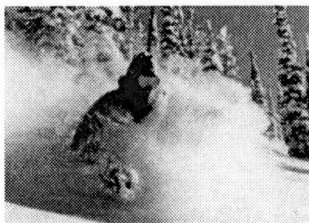

Tip #21: Age is not a barrier

I like to tell clients to stay active and stay young! Building strength and muscle at any age is entirely possible. Numerous landmark studies conclude there is really no difference in the muscle tissue between that of a 30-year-old and a 70-year-old. Biopsies done in laboratory tests showed the muscle tissue of a 70-year-old functions the same as a 30-year-old (*Journal of Applied Physiology*, April 1996). The only difference was in elasticity. Strength was not affected and flexibility dropped a minor degree.

Today, most amateur and professional-level bodybuilding shows are including a growing number of Masters Class body builders who are 40, 50, 60 or more. Olympic greats like Ed Carney, Frank Zane, Robby Robinson, and Bob Parris look as good today as they did twenty years ago. 85-year-old Jack LaLaine is a testament to the power of a lifetime dedicated to fitness. Jack offers $100,000 to any man or woman of any age who can keep up with his daily three-hour workout that involves super-human amounts of aerobics, strength training, calisthenics, swimming, and gymnastics. The editor of *Mens Health* accepted LaLaine's challenge but couldn't stick with him due to nausea. No one has yet to beat Jack the Octogenarian, who clearly has the body and mind of a 30-year-old.

Enhancing functional fitness is another benefit of strength training. Functional fitness is the ability to handle every day tasks with ease and without pain or struggling with injury. These tasks include: walking up stairs, reaching into cabinets, getting in and out of cars, doing housework, lifting grocery bags or kids, handling any calorie-intensive tasks that occur in day-to-day living. Falling is a big issue as people age and occurs because of a lack of strength in the legs and hips. Also, balance and coordination becomes more difficult in advanced age. All these age-related problems have nothing to do with age, but with a lack of activity, exercise, and a decrease in strength that could be alleviated with weight training. The previous thinking that frailty, brittleness, lack of mobility, and slowing down were inevitable products of the aging process are not true. We're finding that less active people are more likely to see these signs of aging while active people retain all the qualities of a youthful body. The message is clear:

STAY ACTIVE!

STAY YOUNG!

LIVE FULLY!

Tip #22: Go for interval training and aerobics to burn fat

Intense bouts of aerobic exercise can be beneficial for men over 40, especially when trying to lose the stubborn INNER TUBE in the stomach area that hides the abs. Remember, the analogy of the charcoal and lighter fluid? This explains how this all works. Just think of your stubborn midsection fat as charcoal, stored fuel waiting to be ignited. As you know it's not easy get charcoal going just as it's not easy to get rid of that fat in your gut. It takes extraordinary measures for your body to use that fat as workout fuel. Unfortunately, men are genetically programmed to hold onto that fat as a survival tool. If you're lost in the wilderness for two weeks, your body will live off the stored fat to keep you alive. The average male stores about 100,000 calories of fat reserves in the body. Science has shown that the best way to tap into that fat (besides a two-week fast) is to shock the body with mild bursts of intense interval aerobic training.

How does it work? If you run on a treadmill for thirty minutes, jack up your intensity by doing one-minute intervals of moderate pace jogging (or walking) and 1 minute intervals of fast running or sprinting or if you're walking, increase the grade and up the speed.

Here's the program some of my clients use:

30 minute interval training
5 minute walking warm-up
1 minute light jogging @ 5.0 m.p.h.
1 minute sprints @ 7.0 m.p.h.
1 minute jogging @ 5.0 m.p.h.
1 minute sprints @ 8.0 m.p.h.
1 minute jog @ 5.0 m.p.h.
1 minute sprint @ 8.5 m.p.h.
1 minute jog @ 5.0 m.p.h.
1 minute sprint @ 9.0 m.p.h.
1 minute jog @ 5.0 m.p.h.

1 minute sprint @ 9.5 m.p.h.
1 minute jog @ 5.0 m.p.h.
1 minute sprint @ 10.0 m.p.h.
1 minute jog @ 5.0 m.p.h.
1 minute sprint @ 10.0 m.p.h.
1 minute jog @ 5.0 m.p.h.
5 minute jog @ 7.0 m.p.h.
5 minute fast walk @ 4.0 m.p.h.

Even the American College of Sports Medicine reversed the institution's official exercise recommendations to say that three- to ten-minute bouts of moderately strenuous activity can be just as beneficial for your cardiovascular health as one 30-minute continuous exercise session. These exercise activities include nothing more strenuous than housework, walking, or gardening, along with more traditional forms of aerobic activity. As mentioned before, this is good news for those people who are just too busy to squeeze in an hour a day. Quick, short and low- intensity does the job just as well as an all-out gut-busting session.

These are great recommendations for baseline fitness but for those of us who need to lose weight or increase our cardio health level we shall need to push the boundary a little further. A good way to start is by taking vigorous walks for a minimum of 30-45 minutes daily. Use some of the many new cardiovascular machines available like the treadmill, the elliptical trainer, the rowing machine, the stair stepper, and the stationary bicycle after you've built up your stamina to do so. Which one is best? The best bang for the buck is the treadmill. It will help you to burn about 25% more calories than all the rest! It's also a good idea to sample different machines and do short 5-10 minutes bouts on a variety of equipment to keep the intensity levels high and the boredom low.

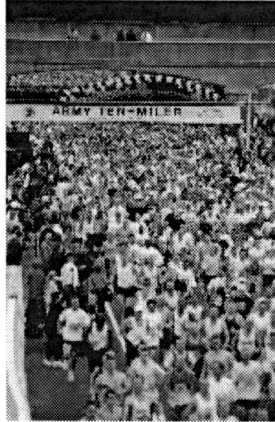

Training, running, walking or biking outdoors has numerous added benefits. The level of difficulty is higher out of doors because of wind resistance, increased need for balancing, and varying grades of hills and terrain that require higher levels of cardio fitness. Working out in cold weather helps you to burn 10% more calories and the scenery is so much more stimulating than a TV Cardio Theater (*source: Strength Coach Charles Polquin*). Fresh air, sunshine, and the adventure of trying new routes make the challenge much more exciting and interesting. Why not enjoy your exercise more and take it outdoors once in a while?

Taking workout shortcuts provides major advantages and allows you to accomplish more in less time:

1. Psychological—you can handle anything in small doses. Facing the daunting task of a 90-minute workout during a busy workday is a daunting task for even the most fanatical and determined. Breaking down the task into smaller, more manageable pieces makes it more appetizing and less unpleasant.

2. Injuries—there is less chance of hurting yourself during shorter workouts and more time for recovery. You allow your body just the right amount of stimulation and exertion followed by a rest period for healing well-used joints, muscles, and tendons.

Below I list a few sample shortcut workouts used by my clients. Remember a shortcut doesn't mean SHORTCHANGE. You are giving yourself better intensity, lowered chance for injury, more free time for your life, and better chance at long-term consistency that gives you a lifetime of good health and a great looking body.

- Supersets, Giant Sets, Triples, Drop Sets
- Hi-rep Strength Circuit/Cardio-Combo Circuits
- Split-Training (one to two body parts per workout)
- Super Slow Training (30-minute session)
- M.A.S.S. (Mature Adult Strength Systems)
- One-Set-to-Failure System
- Strength and Plyometric Calisthenics Combo

Tip #23: Make cardio fun – try something new!

If you prefer to be inside, indoor classes at gyms now offer greater variety than ever. There is a whole new world of "mind-body" fitness like Tai Chi that gives the body and the mind a workout. There are classes that combine disciplines like karate, sports-specific training, and military-style boot camp drills. Here are a few others:

- Jumping rope
- Aqua aerobics
- Urban rebounding (trampoline aerobics)
- Athletic Yoga
- Tae Bo
- Body Pump (aerobics with weights)
- Spinning

New outdoor classes make aerobic exercise interesting and stimulating. Why not join a softball team, play tennis, take up crew, go on long hikes, do biking vacations, enter 5K road races, play volleyball at the beach, go trail biking, or cross country skiing just to name a few.

Tip #24: Train like an athlete in season

Change your thinking about training. Train like an athlete in competition. Enjoyment, fun, and competitive spirit are all aspects of the athlete's mindset. Rather than running the treadmill as punishment for overeating, or bicycling to compensate for missing workouts, begin to look at aerobic training as part of your athletic conditioning. Even if you don't have a sport you can still adopt your favorite exercise to the skill level of a professional athlete. Treadmill running can become an athletic event if you shoot for a 5K race. A stair stepper session can be a practice for mountain climbing or hiking. A stationary bike ride can be good practice for a semi-pro racing team. It can be fun especially if you join a team or group and you can get even better by hiring a coach or trainer who specializes in the particular sport.

Athletes use interval training (also called Fartlek) and speed drills to enhance their skills. These techniques can give some welcome variety to your program. Interval or Fartlek is simply the technique of going fast and then slower at regular timed intervals. Speed drills are measured in time or distance and push your limits of power and endurance in gradual, systematic steps. It's useful to learn these techniques with a sports coach. Find out where your local athletic teams practice and condition during the off- season. Also, if the professional, million-dollar athlete is working out there, it's a safe bet that the facility has high-caliber, well-trained coaches and trainers.

Tip #25: Use gadgets and toys to improve results from training:

Using gadgets is another way to make workouts more effective while keeping training fun and interesting. Heart rate monitors are great for runners and walkers because they help you to get into your optimum fat-burning zone. Many people exercise either too fast or too slow and have problems making progress. Using the monitor shows you exactly how hard you should be exerting yourself to get the maximum return on time invested in aerobic exercise.

The fat burning zone is 60-75% of your maximum heart rate. Exercising in the range provides you the greatest benefit with the least amount of injury. This is a new formula that, according to the *Journal of the American College of Cardiology*, is much more accurate that the industry standard (220, subtract your age and multiply by 70%).

Here's how to find your zone:
[208 – (70% of your AGE)] x .60 [low-end range – 60% of max heart rate]
[208 – (70% of your AGE)] x .75 [high-end range – 75% of max heart rate]

For a typical 48-year-old:
208 – (.70 x 48) = 186.4 x .60 = 111.84
208 – (.70 x 48) = 186.4 x .75 = 130.8

... therefore, 111 is the <u>lowest</u> number in the fat burning zone and 130 is the <u>highest</u> number a 48-year-old would need to get into the fat burning zone.

Using the heart rate monitor on a regular basis will give you an accurate picture of your running or walking intensity. They're available from Polar Company starting at $59.00. Many companies sell some great gadgets online including pedometers, calories trackers, and distance measuring devices.

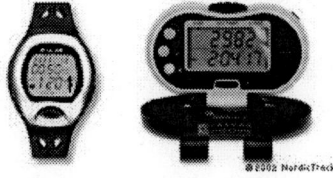

You may also consider getting a professional VO (2) max test done to see how strong your heart and lungs really are. This is the test where you breathe through what resembles a gas mask and have electrodes attached to your chest while you run as fast as possible on a treadmill. A physician then identifies your baseline for monitoring your progress and will show any problems or irregularities with your heart or respiratory system.

<u>Tip #26: Hire a coach or trainer</u>

Another worthy investment is to hire a coach or athletic trainer. You may find your commitment levels increase when you feel accountable to another person for your fitness. The other great benefit is faster improvement and less chance of injury. By putting your financial resources into training you are taking your self-discipline and level of commitment to new and higher levels.

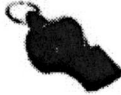

Tip #27: Train for a competitive event

Training for a competition in your sport of choice is perhaps the most exciting, elite, and wonderful place to be. It's challenging and can be grueling but the results and levels of satisfaction reach the pinnacle of experience. Most people get a sense of pride and accomplishment that is unlike anything else they've experienced. The joy of completing a 5K race or being part of a winning team is indescribable. You also get the benefits of developing sport-specific skills, strength for everyday living, a healthy life-enhancing hobby that includes the camaraderie and support of others. A wonderful side effect is weight loss and steady stabilized levels of body fat and higher muscle mass. All in all, the zenith of exercise can be enjoying friendly and/or intense competition!

Another great side effect of aerobics is its anti-aging properties. People who engage in regular aerobic exercise look and actually feel mentally and physically 10 years younger than their non-exercising counterparts. They have more energy, less fatigue and fewer health problems. Aerobics promotes longevity in a new study (see *Runners World*, July 2002).

Tip #28: Use supplements and use them wisely

Here's my trainer secret guide to protein bars, shakes, meal replacement drinks, vitamins, fat burners, and hormones. Most people are justifiably confused and bewildered by the overwhelming choices available to supplement their diets. Many companies' hype, advertising, controversial studies, and the snake oil salesmanship that promote miraculous solutions to fat loss and muscle-building make it difficult to discern what really works from what is a waste of money. In this section, I will serve as your personal Consumer Advocate. This collection of tips will help you make good decisions and right choices that will enhance your goals of fat loss and muscle building. The more educated you are, the better!

Protein Bars and Meal Replacement Powders

When you don't have time to cook or sit down to a full, nutritious meal, protein bars and meal replacement drinks can be a healthy, nutritious alternative. The important thing to remember is that these are REPLACING real food in your eating plan and should absolutely not become your sole source of nutrition. It is always better to eat real food because it contains vitamins, minerals, immune-boosting phytochemicals, fiber, and natural ingredients that are sometimes not present in the more highly processed bars and shakes. If you are faced with a choice of skipping a healthy meal, keep a supply handy and use them with confidence.

A little history: Bars and shakes once were the sole province of hard-core bodybuilders and "fanatical health nuts" until the late 1980s. Most bars and shakes tasted awful, had little nutritional value, and were loaded with sugar, raw egg, and milk powders. The whole industry changed when a young marketing genius named Bill Phillips introduced a product called MetRx™ back in 1990. Physician Scott Connelly developed MetRx™ a nutritious drink that was used to help critically ill people regain their strength and health in a hospital setting.

The drink was revolutionary because it provided the body with high levels of protein and good carbohydrates without being high in calories, sugar, or fat. The protein in this drink was also the most advanced at the time. It had a higher level of "bio availability" which means the body and digestive system processed and used more of the energy in the food itself to be used as fuel for muscle growth and metabolism. The history since has been a series of companies jumping on the bandwagon and mimicking what Bill Phillips did with MetRx™. Since there are so many choices, I advise exercising caution when buying these products. I think the original is still the best and although many have tried to copy the original formula, their products have neither the outstanding taste nor performance.

Snake Oil Scientists

The use of "scientific" claims, non-attributed "clinical" studies, and testimonies from people in the medical field promoting products yielding miraculous results have lessened the image and true value of the good products in the marketplace. There is nothing miraculous or unusual about protein powder. It does not, by itself, make you look like a cover model for *Mens Fitness* (as they would have you believe from the before and after pictures in the glossy magazine ads). The powder is simply a form of nourishment that your body uses to help in the synthesis of repairing muscle tissue after you've had a tough and rigorous strength-training workout. Don't believe everything you read! It's often all hype! A good website to check for accuracy in labeled ingredients is http://www.consumerlab.com.

A super way to see if something works for you is to give a product a fair try. Buy a box and see whether you experience a difference in energy, in how you look, or in how you perform your workouts. You have to be the final judge, because everyone is different and some things work better depending on your individual needs, metabolism, and preferences. Here is my list of the highest quality, high protein/moderate carbohydrate/low fat protein bars. As a general guideline, I look for bars that provide roughly 300 calories, have less than 8 grams of fat or so, and are less than 30 grams of carbohydrates. Each of these bars meets those specifications:

- Pure Protein™ by World Wide Nutrition®
- Protein Revolution™ Bars
- Ultimate Lo Carb™ Bar
- LABRADA Lean Body™ Bar
- Solid Protein™ by Natures Best®
- Designer Whey Protein™ Bar

- Balance™ Bars
- Zone™ Bars
- Luna™ Bars by Clif®
- Premier 8™ by Premier Nutrition®
- Methoxy Pro™ Bar from Cytodyne®
- After FX™ Bar by MetRx®
- Protein Plus™ by MetRx®
- Myoplex Lite™ by EAS®

This is just a small sampler of what is now available. By the time my program is published, new bars will have entered the market.

Here is a list of recommended protein meal replacement powders:

- MetRx Original™
- ULTRAMET™ from Champion Nutrition®
- LEAN BODY™ from LABRADA®
- NUTRIPLEX ™ by Sport Pharma®
- ISO PURE™ from Nature's Best®
- FUEL PLEX™ by Twin Lab®
- APM 60™ by MetRx®
- MYOPLEX Regular™ and Lite Deluxe™ from EAS®
- Designer Whey Protein™
- Veggie Fuel Soy Protein™ by Twin Lab®
- Nitrotech™ by Muscle Tech®
- ProM3™ from ISS Research®
- Promax™ by Sport Pharma®

Some popular product lines that many people use today are fat burners and metabolism boosters. They are also called diet aids, energy boosters, and thermogenic supplements. The common ingredients found in all of them include: caffeine, ma huang, guarana, and ephedrine. There are nervous system stimulants that must be used with caution especially if you have a history of heart disease or stroke in your immediate family take a prescription medicine, have depression, or a mood disorder. The stimulations can be beneficial if used in moderation or on occasion. The "magic" behind these products is that the increase in basal metabolic rate causes a slight increase in fat burning calories and the appetite suppressant creates a calorie deficit that over time causes you to lose weight. Although not scientifically proven, the following diet products are receiving much attention lately and may prove helpful. I recommend using them judiciously and to read the label warnings. Taking them on a daily basis may reduce their effectiveness and increase your health risks. I recommend the following *with strict caution*:

- Yohimbine
- Caffeine/ephedra/willowbark
- Green Tea
- Tyrosine
- L-Carnitine
- HCA
- Synphedrine
- Guggul extract

Popular brands that contain the above ingredients include:

- Ripped Fuel Extreme™ by Twin Lab®
- Xenedrine™
- Thermicore CT™
- Beta Lean™ by EAS®
- Adipokinetix™

Again, try these products at your own risk. They are safe if you take the label recommended dosage, but don't expect to find miracles in a bottle. You must still eat well and follow your exercise plan to get results. These products will give you a boost so you can have a higher intensity workout that may result in a higher number of calories burned and also a higher "after burn effect." Again USE WITH CAUTION AND MODERATION.

Bottled Pre- and Post-workout drinks

The pre-mixed drinks listed are found in most health club vending machines and vitamin and health food stores. Most pre-workout drinks contain stimulants such as ephedrine and caffeine to increase the workout intensity while the post-workout drinks contain a high dose of protein along with carbohydrates to enhance recovery.

If you feel you need a boost before a workout try one and see how it affects you. Remember to be careful if you have hypertension or are taking anti-depressants. Also, stay away from the drinks that have more than 300 calories or those that are exceptionally high in carbohydrates. Post workout drinks should be used with caution also. Choose only those with 20-40+ grams of protein, under 30 grams of carbs and under 300 calories per serving. Because these products are often locally distributed I could not provide an exhaustive list. Read the labels based on the guidelines provided and see which ones work best for you!

Tip #29: Must-have supplements to prevent muscle loss and fat gain

Getting and preserving the hard-earned muscle you've worked so hard to achieve is a tough battle. Your body is constantly in a dynamic state using your muscle tissue as a source of fuel whenever you can't eat at regular intervals or you become stressed, over-trained or physically ill. We want you to preserve your muscles and you can do this through enhancement products.

To help you win the battle against muscle loss, there have been several new products introduced over the past few years that have helped bodybuilders and regular trainees build and retain more muscle. Here is my list of top-quality, proven products you should put on your list to advance toward your fitness goals.

#1 Creatine

Creatine is the most popular and scientifically-proven, effective muscle-builder on the market. The American College of Sports Medicine recommends its use and countless professional athletes, sports teams, and pro body builders use it often. Creatine is effective because it does two things:

a. It increases your muscles' ability to contract with greater strength and explosiveness; and,
b. It fuels the muscle cell with water giving it a swollen appearance that makes your muscles look larger.

Creatine is taken in a loading cycle during the first week. Most manufacturers recommend 20 to 25 grams per day for a full week. Then, clients take a maintenance dose of 5 to 10 grams per day for about two to three months. It is recommended that people go off creatine for a full month and then restart the cycle.

#2 Glutamine

This amino acid is used to build muscle, fuel exercise, enhance the immune system, and to boost brain function and other body systems. A loss of glutamine in the body often occurs from stress, overwork, and strenuous exercise – especially weight training and running. A recent study (*American Journal of Clinical Nutrition*, June 2000) showed that glutamine increased growth hormone 43% in healthy athletes. It also lessens the effects of lactic acid buildup (that pain you feel during the last few reps of an exercise), and boosts the immune system.

#3 ZMA – Zinc Magnesium Aspartate

ZMA helps to maximize your body's anabolic function by increasing levels of free testosterone as well as improving strength, endurance, and muscle recovery.

Here are additional supplements I highly recommend especially for men over 40:

1. A good multi-vitamin
2. Fish oil capsules or Flaxseed oil (UDO's Choice™)
3. Vitamin C in Ester C form
4. Saw palmetto for prostate
5. Glucosamine for joints, tendons, and arthritis
6. Anti-oxidants for immune system protection

Tip #30: Consider the pros and cons of doctor-prescribed testosterone and growth hormones

Pharmaceutical growth hormone (brand name examples: serostim and humatrope) have been on the market for many years to help increase the growth rate of children with slow pituitary glands. A study combined with media hype about the drug's "fountain of youth," anti-aging effects created a new market among Baby Boomers seeking to slow down the aging process. It also became popular with HIV patients experiencing wasting. There was a change in the law regarding growth hormone's use recently and now it is widely available to anyone who wants to use it for health reasons. Bodybuilders have been getting black market and underground versions and swear these hormones have the most powerful effect on muscle growth of all the steroids. I would not recommend this product *unless you are willing* to handle the risks and side effects which include aching joints, acromeglia (a broadening of the forehead), carpal tunnel syndrome, and hypoglycemia. Also growth hormone is expensive—about $1,500 per box!

A whole industry has sprung up from the growth hormone craze. New lines of *growth hormone precursors* have hit the market. Unfortunately, they are not as effective and have a limited effect on natural growth hormone levels. Don't waste your money! Testosterone replacements are also very popular. *Here are the ones currently often promoted*:

- Androstene-dione
- I9-Nora androstene
- 1-Andro diol
- Tirbulus Terrestris
- Tribex 500

All of the above products increase testosterone, but only for a few short hours after they're digested. The effect on muscle growth is minimal, but you must decide for yourself. Try and see if it makes any difference. Most people report marginal change in body composition.

Anabolic steroids – Despite all the numerous benefits, ***it's better to be naturally fit and healthy for life*** instead of building an unhealthy and expensive habit of taking illegal drugs just to look bigger than the next guy. Steroids are non-addictive chemically but the users grow dependent on "the look" and the strength levels, making it hard to come back to normal. Anabolic steroids can be great for men over 40 with low "T" levels. Seek the advice, as always, from your physician.

Looking ahead . . . Anti-aging centers are coming into vogue. Testosterone injections, real growth hormone, and complete supplement regimes are some of the services offered at a new generation of wellness clinics. For men who choose to use steroids, there are institutions staffed by medical doctors who will put you (usually a man over 40 with lower than average testosterone levels) in a complete cycle of steroids, growth hormone, and complementary vitamins and supplement regime based on your goals, lifestyle, and fitness level. Costs vary but most 18-week programs run about $20,000 to $25,000. The jury is still out on the long-term side effects of using steroids and growth for purely aesthetic reasons. This seems to be the wave of the future for those who can afford it. For more information on these treatments, click onto http://www.giovanemed.com.

Engineered Vitamins

A new multi-level marketing gimmick just out on the fitness scene is personalized vitamins and minerals. The promise is a better vitamin suited to your individual metabolism. The user sends a blood sample from a provided kit and the company analyzes the blood, and then sends out the vitamins. Unfortunately, the body can outsmart the vitamins because it will adapt to whatever it is given or for what it is deprived. The human body uses exactly what it needs and disregards the rest. Avoid these engineered products if you are tempted when you see the infomercial. A good multi-vitamin in capsule form is your best bet!

Tip #31: Using herbs can be beneficial

The world of natural medicine has brought a flood of herbal remedies and products into the health food and vitamin shops. There are herbs to prevent, cure, alleviate and soothe almost any physical, mental, or emotional problem. I am not going to spend a lot of time here discussing this vast field, so if you have an interest, I would recommend any of the numerous reference books available in bookstores or online.

Products to avoid:
- Almost any product sold on a TV infomercial, especially pills that promise you can eat all you want and not get fat
- Any product sold in back pages of the *gossip magazines* promising "amazing results in just days"
- Any food supplement that blocks fat or carbohydrate absorption
- Liquid fast diets (where you lose 10 pounds in three days)
- Systems of products from "gurus" or "doctors" promoting miraculous, quick results

Tip #32: One guy's daily regimen – Jim, 44-years-old

Here is an example of a typical day of supplement use from one of my long-term clients, Jim: Jim starts his day off with a breakfast of egg whites and oatmeal, along with a multivitamin, 1 Ester C, 2 glucosamine sulfate capsules for his chronically achy shoulder, and two UDO's Choice Fish Oils™ to supplement his diet and energy needs. At mid-morning he eats a Premier 8™ protein bar along with a large glass of water. Lunch is from the company cafeteria's "healthy selections" – he usually has a big salad with chunks of tuna and a bowl of soup. He forgoes the salad dressing in favor of a tablespoon of parmesan cheese and a splash of vinegar.

By mid-afternoon Jim is starting to get a little hungry again so he goes to the office kitchenette and eats a small 8-ounce container of nonfat cottage cheese with Splenda™ sweetener. He always keeps a stash of snacks in the office fridge like fresh fruit, nonfat fruit yogurt, smoked salmon, and pre-cooked chicken breast.

After work, Jim heads right to his health club. While dressing he eats a small Balance Bar™ to fuel his workout and keep up his energy. Next, on his way home from the gym he stops at a neighborhood catering market and buys a half rotisserie chicken, steamed vegetables, and fresh fruit medley. Within an hour of finishing his workout he is sitting down to a healthy meal, relaxing with his dog in front of the fireplace. The grueling leg routine really knocked him out and it's just good to sit and relax with a book. About an hour before bed Jim mixes up his favorite snack, vanilla pudding made with MetRx™ protein powder. This gives his muscles enough protein and nourishment as they begin the long process of rebuilding and recovering during the night.

Tip #33: Techniques for making better fat-burning choices

Here are some sure-fire solutions for getting through the tough times of temptation. Use these techniques and separate yourself from the talkers and daydreamers who are always going on and off diets and exercise programs. These suggestions are proven to help you win the battle of the bulge and reach your goal body.

1. ***Practice Saying No.*** No matter what the situation, you always have a choice. Empower yourself by saying, "No thank you, I rather not eat that right now. My hard-earned washboard abs and muscular definition are not worth a piece of cheesecake or a pint of Haagen-Dazs."

2. ***Always ask yourself, "What is my MOTIVATION for reaching this weight loss goal?"*** The clearer the picture of what you see as the end result, the easier it is to make the right choices that move you towards your goal. You'll be far more motivated to continue and forge ahead when the going gets tough if you:

   a. Have a written date or deadline for the goal;

   b. Have a "fridge pic" of what you believe you can look like;

   c. Have a person or role model that you emulate such as a person who has reached the pinnacle with your body type; and,

   d. Have a written "Presume" – a story that presumes you are 1 year into the completion of a goal and tells the story in vivid detail of how it happened. Write as if your goal is a part of your past history and are reminiscing about how you got to where you finally wanted to be (see page XX for more details).

TIP #34: <u>Use affirmations and personal mantras</u>

The following can help to remind you when you start down the slippery slope of overeating, bingeing or emotional eating. Here are some of my clients' personal favorites:

a. "I can have more later on. On this diet I eat every 2 ½ to 3 hours. I can wait a little longer to eat. I don't need to finish this all right now."

b. "I make *better* bad choices when *ideal* is not available to me."

c. "If you wanna be ripped, don't let it hit the lips."

d. "My wants are not my needs. I need real nourishment from food and not ice cream, for survival and healthy well-being."

e. "I am eating everything I need to reach my goal of muscular definition and washboard abs."

f. "Green is lean; white is light."

g. "A craving is only a feeling – it will pass."

h. "Thin tastes better."

i. Ask yourself, "Do you like that enough to wear it on your abs, hips, and waist?"

j. "You can't have everything you want, but you always get what you need."

k. "You've come too far in life to take orders from a cookie."

l. "No forbidden foods – only forbidden ways of eating them."

m. "Planning is stronger than willpower. Be armed and ready, shop healthy, cook healthy."

n. "Every time I say 'No, thank you,' I say yes to the body I want!"

The most difficult part of your new eating program phases in after the first month when the initial enthusiasm passes and some of the old habits creep back. You need to stay motivated by pumping yourself up on a daily basis. You can use "medicine chest affirmations." Write-up personal affirmations on small index cards and tape them onto your bathroom mirror or inside your medicine chest. What are personal affirmations? Affirmations are things you say to yourself in a positive, emotionally enthusiastic way that reinforce your goal or desired outcome. They are always stated in the present tense as if they were really happening. These don't necessarily have to be true at the time but by feeding these to your subconscious on a regular basis, it leads you to people, places, situations, and circumstances that support you and help you to move ahead and be where you want to be.

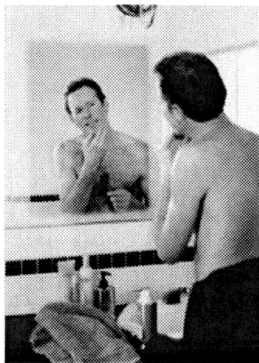

Here are some of my favorites:

1. "I can eat more later on; I don't need to eat it all now."

2. "I eat everything I need today to maintain a muscular, well-defined body."

3. "Today I get the help I need from others to support my efforts at weight loss."

4. "I am able to choose the foods that make me lean and I reject the types and quantities of food that make me fat."

5. "I do whatever it takes to get my workout done today."

Here is one of my all time favorites:

"There is no obstacle, no situation or problem that can circumvent, hinder, or otherwise control the firm resolve of a determined soul like me to make a change in my habits or reach a goal. I do whatever it takes and I keep at it until I am successful regardless of setbacks or disappointments." The above quote is taken from Hyrum W. Smith's 1994 book Ten Natural Laws of Successful Time and Life.

Tip #35: Follow the "rule of half"

Remember: Your new body begins in the supermarket when you recognize the conditioned cravings and temptations, but do not give into them. Eat half of what you were craving and see if it satisfies. Then eat, share it, or throw it out. Can you substitute for something lower in fat or calories to satisfy your craving? Many chocoholics find great satisfaction with chocolate protein bars, or chocolate protein drinks rather than emptying an 8 oz. bag of M&Ms™.

Personal Trainer Secrets: numerous scientific studies have shown there is no physiological, biological, or chemical basis for cravings (source: LEARN program from Dr. Kelly Brownell). Cravings are mostly brought on by environmental factors such as television commercials, visual, and olfactory cues, (walking by a steak shop or Chinese restaurant on the way home from work can cause a craving for fatty foods). Shopping mall food courts are strategically located to tempt us with the smells of fresh and hot muffins, cookies, and fast food such as KFC® or McDonalds®.

Don't give into "all or nothing" mentality when you've blown a meal. Just take a cue from the ancient Greeks: practice moderation.

Tip #36: Act like a practicing Buddhist – take the middle way

Go to neither extreme. Use the driving analogy. Stay focused on the road ahead. When you veer off to the right or left, steer back to the middle. Make adjustments along the way, but don't kick yourself and crash the car just because you've veered off for a few seconds. Giving up on your eating program is equivalent to letting the car go off the road into a ditch and rollover. Remember, one meal does not make you fat – DON'T DESPAIR!

Tip #37: Delay gratification

- Set a kitchen timer for 15 minutes, and get busy – see if it doesn't work
- Go for a 15-minute walk
- Distract yourself with something not food-related
- Have sex
- Go shopping for your new, thinner wardrobe
- Look at exercise machines – pictures and articles strengthen good behaviors
- Drink a large glass of water

Use the battle analogy to break cravings and binges. Always arm yourself with the good foods you know will help you reach your goals. Re-supply your munitions of fruit, veggies, lean fish, and meat at a weekly scheduled time. Remain constantly vigilant and alert to the traps, pitfalls, and land mines that trigger your poor eating patterns. Know your enemy and how it operates. Fight for your freedom from fat and from old enslaving habits.

Tip #38: Handle cravings as you would a two-year-old

When cravings for junk food hit, visualize them as spoiled little two-year-olds jumping up and down pleading and provoking, crying, and screaming for candy. Do you give in to the taunts and cries of the little devil? Do you try to scold or ignore him? Can you soothe the two-year-old with love, attention, and compassion. Try to play the adult role when your two-year-old tantrum-maker interferes with your peace of mind and your goals. Stand your ground, be firm, do what's good for the child in the long run. If he won't cut back his whining, put him in his room until he stops. Who's in control? Who has the authority and the power in this situation?

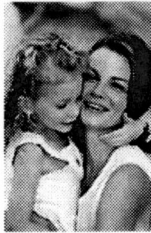

Tip #39: Borrow techniques from AA

In the AA program there is a recognizable phrase that explains the reasons for drinking: It's all about **people, places, and things**. The reasons for most bad or self- destructive behavior stem from how you react to the people, places, and things in your life. That's why AA members are encouraged to socialize, do business with, and to 'just hang out' with one another to support a common goal. In the same way you can also help yourself by being with others who support your healthy eating and exercise lifestyle. Drop your friends from the nightly wine and cheese connoisseurs club! Hang around more with others who are in the same fitness and eating program. Socialize with others who are already successful and living the lifestyle. Seek out the winners who are doing what you are striving for and become one, too!

Alcoholics Anonymous has some fantastic, inspirational quotes that can help you weather any difficult storm:

a. "This too shall pass."
b. "Let go, let God."
c. The Serenity Prayer: "God grant me the serenity and courage to change the things I can, accept the things I can't change, and the wisdom to know the difference."

Tip #40: Master tough food choices in social situations

Now, imagine the scenario: you are going to a company cocktail reception, surrounded by people you don't really want to be with (you might wish you could stay home and rent a movie) but it's an obligation you just can't avoid! To occupy your time at the party, you spend time hovering around the buffet table, nervously nibbling on everything in sight. There are many unhealthy food choices and lots of goodies you really like. The sweet table is loaded with cookies and petit fours. Don't give up just yet! Take my advice and do the following:

- Eat 1/3 less calories at every meal you have on this day from breakfast through lunch and snacks;
- Count this specific event as one of your splurge meals;
- Plan on staying at the event briefly – an hour or two at most;
- Reach out and engage in conversation one stranger at the party; and,
- Plan your calorie strategy. Eat the things your really, really love – only those things that are truly worth the calories. If you're a dessert lover, skip the hors'd'ouvres and the mediocre entrées (or eat ½ the entrée), double-up on salad and vegetables and then enjoy a dessert without worry.

An awkward situation: When you're eating in someone's home, and they insist that you have seconds or extra large portions, you can fib. Fake an allergy, say you have intestinal distress, or explain that you cannot operate too much rich food. Tell them you're on a special lifesaving cholesterol lowering diet. If they insist you eat dessert when you're full, tell them you're a recently diagnosed insulin-sensitive hypoglycemic. If all else fails, just ask for a miserly portion and eat a small amount and stop (then maybe give the rest to the dog!).

Tip #41: Learn the dirty little secret of the most successful dieters . . . PORTION CONTROL

Portion control is all about setting boundaries on the foods you love and the ones you need for good nutrition and slow steady fat loss. Why are Lean Cuisine®, Weight Watchers®, and Healthy Choice® frozen entrées so successful? There is nothing magical or mysterious in the ingredients. Many of them are made with heavy starches and fats (which is why they taste so great). Lean Cuisine® has a delicious macaroni and cheese dish. Examine closely the label and see that there's nothing intrinsically or exceedingly healthy about it. The true secret to their miniscule calorie count is the portion size and packaging. The picture on the package is actually larger than the food inside the box.

The great advantage to using these products is that you can eat the foods you love (some forbidden treats) and still stay within a reasonable daily calorie range. I recommend these to all my clients if they have trouble with overeating or have poor judgment in either overestimating or underestimating the amount of food they consume. Serve them with a big green salad or a bowl of assorted cooked vegetables, add fruit and yogurt for dessert, and you've got an ideal meal.

Tip #42: Know thyself

We all have histories with certain kinds of foods that lead us down the path to temptation and possible relapse. It is important _to know thyself_. Recognize your difficult areas and the bad food magnets or trigger foods. All the willpower in the world will not prevent a chocoholic from eating the Godiva® chocolates he brought home from the company party. [**An important note**: Don't sabotage your efforts by bringing tempting foods into the house in the first place. Clean out your cupboards and fridge from temptations.] For example, avoid restaurants where you have a fetish for their New York style cheesecake or banana split sundae. You might even consider rerouting your way to work to avoid that bakery where you used to purchase those 500 calorie muffins. Most muffins are 25% (and upwards) of your daily caloric intake! Don't allow yourself to get so hungry that you can't wait to eat everything in sight.

Tip #43: Willpower is useless in the long haul – here's what some of my clients have done

Smart planning works; willpower doesn't work alone in a vacuum. Acknowledge that you can feel powerless in certain food-related situations. You can butt heads and get mad as hell, but the food gremlins will always return to haunt you. The best thing to do is to acknowledge the habit, accept it, and honor it as part of your personality that served a purpose at one time but now is no longer valid.

Einstein once said, "You cannot solve a problem with the same mind that created it." You need to replace one habit with another. Your desire for chocolate chip cookies at 11:00 p.m. can be replaced by eating fat-free, low sugar chocolate frozen yogurt. Find a good substitute or change the situation that brings on the cravings, urges, and food obsessions. Instead of watching TV and eating, plan an evening out, volunteer, train for a new sport, or try a new hobby. Go out and walk for an hour on a new route. Call an old friend, meditate, listen to beautiful music or net surf and expand your knowledge. You do have choices, you have the power to make a change – you just need to use your head and believe wholeheartedly that it will happen.

Weight Loss Winners Share their Secrets

Here are some strategies my clients and friends employed to successfully lose and maintain their weight. It's tough keeping the weight off when things start to get tough and resolve crumbles. The following case studies illustrate what worked over the years and how clients maintained successful weight loss and eating lifestyle changes.

Paul F. ➔ "When I feel a food urge or a need to binge I remind myself of how far I've come. The fear of going back to the beginning scares me and *that's enough* to motivate me and help me take control."

Perry M., age 33 ➔ "I recall one winter when I did not fit into my clothes. When I was traveling a ton for work I kinda porked out. Now that

78

I'm back into shape, I find some motivation from various things. One of my tricks is to visualize the picture of the guy I taped to the outside of my refrigerator. This guy has total washboard abs and well-defined pecs. If I keep the picture of the goal in front of me, I feel I can't fail."

Kevin➜ "Knowing I have to write down my food and then show it to my trainer makes me think twice about overindulgence. Being accountable to someone else has made all the difference."

Darren F., age 31 ➜ "I don't want to blow all the hard work. One of my coping methods when faced with junk foods is just to taste, but not even come close to finishing the junk food in front of me."

George W, age 52 ➜ "Swear off personal 'trigger foods' – the ones you cannot eat just one of like cookies or chips."

Joe M., age 71 ➜ "A regular walk/job routine combined with weight training is an effective way of reducing fat levels. I walk for a minute, jog for a minute to keep my heart rate in the fat-burning zone four times a week and then on intervening days strength train with free weights."

Ryan V., age 40 ➜ "Twenty minutes of cardio in the morning and small meals every three hours works wonders for me."

Dennis R., age 41 ➜ "Tell everyone what your goal is and when you hope to achieve it. I have shared this simple tip with several friends and they love to hate it! They love it because they achieve all their goals, but hate it because they are constantly reminded of their commitments forcing them into the gym, onto the running track, and away from the kitchen table. I have lost an incredible 36 pounds and dropped five inches from my waist. My entire motivation comes from this one small tip. It's simple and it works."

James K., age 63 ➜ "I eat no more than I burn. I generally try to avoid junk food but am not overly strict with my diet, or I couldn't stick to it day after day. I eat really well during the week, then splurge on the weekends with a nice restaurant meal."

Phil C., age 53 ➜ "My best results come from sprints. I do 100% all out intensity for just 30 seconds while running or cycling, then drop down to about half of that and do a slow jog for a minute. I usually repeat this six or seven times for a good fat-burning workout."

Christopher R., age 47 ➜ "Cut out processed foods which contain high amounts of sugar, sodium, and white flour that your body simply doesn't need. In addition to cutting up and looking more muscular, I have more energy when I switch from processed to fresh foods."

Jerry K., age 43 ➜ "Change your routines periodically – monthly with weights and every other week with cardio. This keeps your muscles growing and prevents your body from growing accustomed to your exercises. This simple method has helped me lose 45 lbs and reduce my body fat from 28% to 12%."

John B., age 59 ➜ "I just say NO to junk food. I lost 30 lbs by refusing to buy any more ice cream and Pepperidge Farm cookies. I made a determined effort to cut them out of my diet and it really worked. I began eating smaller portions of healthier foods and after several months lost an additional 25 lbs. I do a regular weight routine and run and bike for aerobic activity. It feels great not hauling around an extra 55 lbs of blubber."

Jim C., age 51 ➜ "I was once 250 lbs and only 5'6". I started running every morning before breakfast. I didn't see results right away, but after I mixed in weight training with the running, the weight just started to pour off. That's when I started to hear the "wow, you're losing weight!" comments from friends and co-workers. I do a 30-minute run five days a week and weight train every other day. I avoid fast food and never bring junk food into my house. I'm now a lean 170 lbs, a weight I haven't seen since high school."

David B ➜ "I run before breakfast. This creates a fitness mentality I hold onto the rest of the day, helping me to eat healthier and exercise more. I drink more liquids than I used to (mostly water and diet soda). This seems to fill me up and temporarily subdue my hunger pangs."

Peter W., age 67 ➜ "I keep inspirational notes on my refrigerator such as 'Nothing tastes as good as being thin.'"

Jeff R., age 49 ➜ "The single most effective method for fat loss is high intensity resistance and cardio work and especially circuit training."

Dominic H., age 50 ➜ "Seeing young men who look years older than me is a great motivator."

Alan S., age 45 ➜ "I make lunch hour on Monday, Wednesday, and Friday my workout time. If someone wants to schedule something for those times, I'll say, 'Sorry, I'm booked then.'"

Josh M., age 40 ➜ "A little planning goes a long way. On Sunday morning I cook and prepare a week's worth of lunches and snacks for work. I have no excuse for not eating right while at work."

Jeff S., age 51 ➜ "I think about how much better I feel when I'm finished with a workout. I realize that workouts don't have to be all or nothing. When I don't feel like exercising, I just decrease the intensity. It's better to do something than nothing at all."

Barry J., age 43 ➜ "Working out has become my personal time. Those few hours at the gym each week times when I can focus on nothing else but myself. No problems, no worries, just me and the weights. That's where I can make my own personal goals happen."

Tom Z. ➜ "I'd go crazy without any junk food so I treated myself to 200 empty calories a day, either an ice cream sandwich (about 190 calories, or 3-4 pieces of bite-size chocolates). For me, it worked. I never binged and lost the weight."

Tip #44: How to eat healthfully when you're not home

Here are some tough situations you will encounter while eating away from home:
1. Restaurants
2. Parties in an office, home, or outdoor setting
3. Weddings, banquets – the major life events
4. Sporting events
5. Driving for vacation, pleasure, or business or just getting around town
6. Dinner at Mom's, relatives' or at the home of a gourmet food enthusiast

Remember no matter what the situation, if you believe you have control and can positively visualize yourself handling the most difficult of temptations by just saying, "No, thank you," you will have developed the most noble of qualities that eludes most people – self-discipline. Having self-discipline is just a form of self-control that I call "won't power." It **WORKS** much better than will power. You have the power to say **NO**. Try it and practice it right now. Say "No" out loud and feel how it empowers you.

We're so used to compromising to please others and afraid of hurting others' feelings. Be selfish for a change, look out for your own best interests. **Say NO to food you don't need, and see how good it makes you feel.**

Let's look at each situation and see how easy it can be to do the right things. *Restaurants are the #1 killer of diets and there are several reasons*:
1. The portions are often two to three times too large
2. The food is usually enhanced with hidden fats. Butter, oil, and cheese are the things that make restaurant food so good.
3. Menus are deceptive and the wording doesn't give an ordinary person clues as to how healthy or fattening a dish will be.

KITCHEN CONFIDENTIAL

The best strategy for ordering at restaurants regardless of their ethnic origin, price range, or reputation is very simple:
1. Ask how much fat, oil, or butter is used in the dish.
2. Avoid sauces or ask for them on the side. Tomato sauce is usually a safe choice. Broiled doesn't mean healthy, unless you ask for the item dry, without butter.
3. Go for grilled items to minimize fat and maximize flavor.
4. Ask for double the vegetables and omit the starch. Potatoes, rice, and pastas are loaded with butter and oil to keep them from drying out in the hot restaurant kitchen steam table.
5. Go for white chicken, whitefish, pork tenderloin, alligator, veal, tofu, turkey, poultry and shellfish. Those choices are always lower in calories than dark meats. Plus, venison, ostrich, buffalo and most wild game meats make outstanding choices.
6. Order salads with dressing on the side. Dip the tines of your fork in the dressing and then spear the salad greens. You can also ask for low fat salad dressing.

If you must splurge on dessert, go for something non-creamy and split it with your dining companions, or just eat three to four bites. If you want to cut an additional 300 to 500 calories off the meal, just refuse the bread and butter basket. Order soup as an appetizer. It's filling and nutritious. Don't be afraid to make a special request of your server. Tell them you are on a low fat diet and ask them for suggestions. Sometimes they will be helpful but many wait staff are not trained in suggesting the most nutritional and healthy food suggestions to their guests. So be prepared and use the suggestions above to make the choices that will keep you on track and win the battle of the bulge.

Best choices at selected restaurant types for eating healthfully:
1. **Diners** – Order broiled, dry fish and double the vegetables. Or, order an egg white omelette with tomato and spinach and replace the bread and/or potatoes with either fresh greens or another vegetable.

2. **Italian** – Order grilled, thin veal cutlets (not breaded), ask for the salad dressing on the side, choose minestrone soup, and pick the items with red sauce. Avoid the pastas and cannollis for dessert

3. **Chinese** – A dangerous diet dilemma, but you can order soup for an appetizer, ask for a no oil stir-fry chicken and vegetables, and eat 1/3 of the rice they give you. Ask for ½ of your entrée to be wrapped and enjoy it for lunch or dinner the next day! One fortune cookie is okay; these treats mostly consist of sugar and egg whites.

4. **Salad Bars** – Often a great choice. Just watch out for fat or sugar-laden dressings.

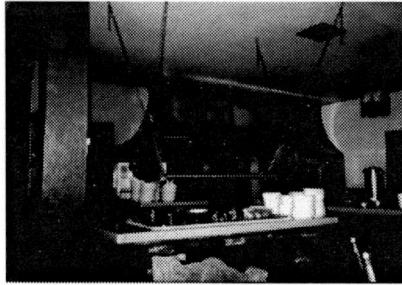

5. **Japanese** – Sushi and sashimi restaurants are great bets with their high protein, moderate carbs, and very low fat dishes. If you don't like raw fish, the teriyaki grilled chicken or fish is very low in fat and comes with a vinaigrette salad that makes an ideal combination.

6. **Middle Eastern** – Turkish, Lebanese, and Greek foods are very similar and can be very healthy if you order carefully. The cuisine is based on whole grains, yogurt, fresh vegetables, and grilled meats (kebobs). Be careful with hummus and pita bread (the hummus is very high in fat) and forgo the Baklava desserts that are very calorie-dense.

7. **Steakhouses** – Order the smallest filet on the menu (four to six ounces) or choose grilled chicken, fish, or pork without sauce. Order an a la carte side of broccoli or (any plain steamed vegetable) and eat only half the starch. Shrimp or crab cocktail is a good choice for an appetizer. Avoid the bread and desserts.

8. *Ethnic cuisine to avoid <u>except on splurge days</u>* – English,

French, Irish, Scottish, Indian, Mexican, German, Scandinavian, Eastern European (Russian, Ukrainian, Polish), traditional African-American "soul food", and home style Latin foods.

Tip #45: Simplify shopping

Here are some useful shortcuts to help make food shopping quick and easy. Everyone has time limitations and the sooner and more efficiently you get this done, the more time you'll have for the important things in life.

The key to success in any eating program begins with planning. Planning is stronger than will power. A clear game plan of what you'll eat for the coming week gives you an advantage that will help you through difficult days when the last thing you need to think about is food preparation. When you have determined the number of calories you need and selected your menu of **TOP 15** favorite foods, the next thing is to make a list and go to your favorite supermarket. Hopefully, the store you select is fairly close to home and will carry a wide range of items, especially fresh produce, fish, and meats. Farmers markets are great alternatives for finding fresher and more exotic varieties of fruits and vegetables. Ethnic markets in the larger cities carry a bevy of healthy foods and give you a chance to experiment with new tastes and textures in food.

The shopping list is a <u>BLUEPRINT FOR SUCCESS</u>. I always tell my clients the first line of defense against breaking poor eating habits is the supermarket. Because the majority of food you consume will likely be prepared and eaten at home, or packed and taken with you, it is essential to become familiar with the supermarket in which you feel most comfortable. Working from a list is vital. When you have a list there's less temptation to deviate. You may not feel swayed to try all the goodies on the end displays or by the double coupon sales (or the Double-Stuff Oreos™ for that matter). Spend about five minutes reviewing your breakfast, lunch, dinner, and snack needs and then write them down on a small index card. Create columns for each of the following items: Fruits & Vegetables[1], Frozen Goods[2], Dairy/Meat/Fish[3], Canned Goods/Dry Goods[4] and Snacks/Condiments[5].

Keep the card in your kitchen throughout the week and jot down items as you finish them off. This is especially good to do on items that are part of your basic cupboard stock spices, condiments, canned goods, coffee, beverages, etcetera. Pick a time of day to go shopping when you are the least bit hungry. Don't go when your hunger pangs are rolling. You are more likely to purchase items that are bad choices for fitness. Always shop **AFTER** you've eaten to avoid giving in to hunger temptations.

Getting the Basics

My mantra for the healthy eating lifestyle – ARM YOURSELF WITH GOOD FOOD CHOICES AT HOME. Guard yourself against the onslaught of daily temptation and uncontrollable food lust by having readily available and accessible selections of tasty, appealing foods in your kitchen.

The first thing I do with my clients is to go through their kitchens and help them clear out the temptations. Empty the pantry of high fat crackers, snacks, cookies, last year's fruit cake, canned cake frosting, Crisco™, canned foie gras, or whatever calorie-dense food you have that may cause problems down the road.

Go through the refrigerator and clear the shelves of high fat, high sugar foods. Toss out the Godiva™ gift box, the old wheel of brie, the canned soda, frozen birthday cake, and the leftover Dominos© Pizza. Toss or donate all foods outside of your new eating plan.

One of the best ways to assure success in eating at home is to have an **OVERABUNDANCE** of healthy items to choose from. In the world of coaching, we call this Creating a SUPER-RESERVE. Simply having just enough is **not** going to be **good enough** for you. You will need to have a constant, steady supply of all the food and supplements that will help you reach your bodily goals and enjoy life with good food. In fact, just as an exercise, the first few weeks I want you to buy more than you think you'll need to keep your kitchen stocked. Having a super-reserve on hand helps during busy weeks when going food shopping is a low priority. For example, I always keep my cabinets full of canned tuna (in water, not oil, of course), canned soup, and assorted varieties of hot cereals like oatmeal. If I miss food shopping that week I can make healthy meals from those items in a matter of minutes. It doesn't allow you to come home and say, "There's nothing to eat, so, I'll just call for pizza."

One of the biggest reasons I hear for diet failure is "I ran out of food because I couldn't get to the store this week. That's why I ordered the Chinese food that came with the free fried egg roll and fried rice." I know these little tricks that our minds can play on ourselves all too well. Building a Super-Reserve of good foods supports your lifestyle and helps you avoid

Jim Hart, A.C.E.

the failure set-up of *RAVAGING-HUNGER-AND-NOTHING-IN-THE-HOUSE* SYNDROME.

Here are the most important items to have in your kitchen cabinets:

Condiments & Prepared Foods

- A wide variety of spices from multiple ethnic traditions
- Sea salt, kosher salt, low sodium salt
- Non-fat salad dressings
- Non-fat mayonnaise
- Salsa – all varieties (non-fat without oil)
- Ketchup – try exotic plum, ginger, or hot brands
- Relish/chutney/barbeque sauce
- Pickles (careful if you are watching your sodium)
- Flavored vinegars, aged balsamic vinegar
- Sugar-free syrups, Splenda™, Sweet & Low™
- Marinades, bottled sauces
- Wonder Butter™ low-fat peanut butter

Grains & Cereals

- Shredded Wheat™
- Rice cakes, corn cakes
- Oatmeal, regular, Irish, steel cut (long cooking)
- Cream of rye, barley, rice or multi-grain mix
- Grits, cornmeal
- Brown rice
- Kashi cereal, all cold and hot versions
- Quinoa, amaranth (exotic grains from health food store)
- All-bran™, extra fiber cereal
- Fiber One™ bran cereal
- Wheat germ
- Unprocessed raw wheat bran and oat bran
- TVP – textured vegetable protein (soy protein nuggets are similar to grape nuts in texture)

- Puffed rice
- Uncle Sam's™ cereal
- Puffed wheat
- Wheetabix™ cereal
- Low-carb pancake mix, bread mix
- Whole wheat pasta, low-carb pasta
- Soy pasta and macaroni
- Buckwheat noodles
- Whole grain breads
- Low-carb soy breads
- Whole grain English muffins

Canned Goods

- Tuna, salmon, crab, shrimp, sardines, squid, clams, oysters, and anchovies
- Fat free chili, stews
- All varieties of non creamy soups (Healthy Choice™ & Campbell's Healthy Request™)
- Chicken broth
- Canned tomatoes and stewed, chopped, pureed tomato sauce (use Ragu Lite™, Healthy Choice™, or any brand under 50 calories per ½ cup
- Canned vegetables (asparagus, green beans, spinach)
- Canned chicken, turkey
- Italian marinated vegetables in vinegar (giardinera, red peppers, sweet peppers, cherry peppers)
- All varieties of beans especially garbanzo, lentils, soy, black, pigeon peas, lima, navy, and red kidney

Beverages

- Spring water
- Crystal Lite™
- Diet soda

- Coffee, tea, green tea, herbal tea
- Skim milk
- Tomato, V8™ juice
- Low sugar, or sugar-free juice drinks
- Sugar-free iced tea mix
- Sugar-free, fat-free hot chocolate

Stock Your Refrigerator & Freezer

- Meats, poultry, game
- Boneless chicken
- 95% lean ground beef
- Ground turkey breast (white breast meat under 2% fat)
- Turkey cutlets
- Top or bottom round of beef
- Filet mignon (3 ounce portions)
- Pork tenderloin or boneless chops
- Venison, ostrich, boar, or buffalo (super-lean red meats)

Seafood

- Frozen tuna burgers and salmon burgers
- All varieties of white fish (flounder, cod, striped bass, mahi-mahi')
- All varieties of shellfish (crab, lobster, shrimp, clams, mussels, squid)
- Oily fish (salmon, swordfish, bluefish)
- Take-home sushi
- Fake crab meat ("Surimi")
- Moderate oil fish such as tuna, striped bass, cod, steelhead trout, shark, catfish
- Cured or smoked salmon (and most varieties of smoked fish)
- Pickled herring/gifilte fish

Dairy

- Eggs
- Egg Beaters™ & pasteurized egg whites
- Non-fat or very low-fat cheese
- Smart Squeeze™ liquid butter substitute
- Low-fat spread able butter or margarine products (search for brands less than 5 g fat/serving such as Benecol™)
- Non-fat cottage cheese or 1% cottage cheese
- Yogurt (light varieties about 120 calories per cup)
- Sour cream (non-fat)
- Soy cheese
- Farmers cheese
- Non-fat ricotta cheese
- Low-fat feta cheese
- Parmesan (under 1 g fat/tablespoon)
- Pre-shredded (low-fat or nonfat) bagged cheese, especially mozzarella, cheddar, Swiss, and Monterrey Jack

Fruit

All varieties are recommended. Be sure to buy fresh, in-season fruit and try something new and exciting if it looks interesting. Frozen berries are a great taste of summer during the cold weather months.

Vegetables – Frozen & Fresh

All varieties of frozen and fresh vegetables are recommended. You can eat as much as you want. Fresh salad greens or pre-bagged salad mixes make a great addition to your must-have collection. A guilt-free, low calorie all-you-can-eat-choice!

Vegetables – Starches

We should exercise caution with starchy vegetables and monitor our portion sizes as starchy vegetables are three times as calorie dense as the fibrous veggies mentioned above.

- Potatoes (all varieties, especially red, purple, and Yukon gold)
- Yams
- Sweet potatoes
- Lima beans
- Soy beans
- Chick peas
- Corn
- Peas
- Sugar snap peas
- Lentils
- Succotash
- Rice – brown and wild

Frozen Convenience Foods

- Lean Cuisine™
- Health Choice™
- Weight Watchers™ dinners
- Mrs. Paul's™ grilled fish filets (about 100 calories each)
- Mrs. Paul's Healthy Selects™ baked fish filets and fish sticks
- Purdue Shortcuts™ cooked chicken
- Veggie burgers (all varieties)
- Fat-free hot dogs & sauerkraut
- Banquet™ Fat-free baked chicken cutlets

Snacks

- *#1 Favorite*: Glenny's Soy Crisps™ (low fat, high protein, low carb, low cal)

- Jell-O™ sugar-free, fat-free pudding and gelatin mixes
- Guiltless Gourmet™ fat-free bean dip
- Jerky: beef, ostrich, turkey, vegetarian
- Finn Crisp™ crackers
- Wasa Crisp™ breads
- Pickled eggs (whites only)
- Soy snack chips, veggie chips
- Baked corn tortillas
- Popcorn (Healthy Choice™)
- Non or low-fat potato chips (single portion)
- Single portion bags of pretzels, soy nuts

Remember you are facing a battle against old habits. Your kitchen is the battleground where you must be armed and ready with healthy food choices that support your new lifestyle and super-fit body. Your ammunition against overeating when you come home tired, frustrated and exhausted from working all day are the cabinets and refrigerator shelves filled with fresh vegetables, lean protein, and light dairy snacks. Don't be caught by surprise by not preparing a shopping list and going to the store at least once a week to stock up. The enemy is lurking – be on the lookout and be vigilant. Your victory is assured and the body you want is guaranteed if you follow these guidelines.

Tip #46: Do a kitchen makeover

One of the best ways to be successful in your new program is to re-do your kitchen by stocking it with all the items, tools, and foods that will guarantee your success. Getting rid of temptations is Job #1 during the kitchen makeover. I love doing this with my clients; it's an educational experience and gets them off to a good start. I always schedule this the weekend before they begin their new eating plan and just before the first big shopping trip.

Here's how we do it:
1. Set a date and time for the kitchen makeover when you know that you will not be interrupted.
2. Tackle the cupboards, pantry, and refrigerator individually.
3. Read the ingredients and calorie counts of every product you have and ask, "Will this support me in my goal of eating for muscular definition and fat loss?"
4. Keep a running list of items you will need to replace when you go shopping.
5. Keep garbage bags handy. Throw away or donate foods that don't support your goals.

Foods to get rid of in your pantry and cupboard:
- High sugar cereal
- Highly processed canned goods
- Creamy soups
- Spam™ or deviled ham
- Oil-packed tuna
- Vegetable oil or Crisco™
- White flour starches, egg noodles, white rice
- Snack foods, chips, puffs, pretzels, etc.
- White bread/muffins/bagels
- Candy/crackers/cookies
- Full-fat mayonnaise/salad dressings
- Honey/white sugar/maple syrup

- Sweet pickles and sweet mustards
- Sugary condiments and ice cream toppings
- Any item with high amounts of fructose or corn syrup

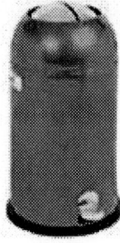

Foods to remove from your refrigerator and freezer:
- Canned fruit in heavy syrup
- Sugar-sweetened juices
- Full-fat dairy products, cheese, yogurt, milk
- Processed meats, sausages, pepperoni, lunchmeat
- Margarine, butter, whipped cream, canned cheese
- Peanut butter with added oil and sugar
- Jams and jellies
- High-fat cuts of beef, ground dark meat turkey
- Smoked meats
- Frozen desserts, ice cream, sweet treats

How to Make Your Kitchen a Better Place

Here is a checklist of "must-haves" to make your kitchen an easier, more efficient place to cook and prepare quick nutritious meals and snacks:

Microwave

Indoor grill (like the George Forman™) or sauté pan with grill surface

Professional chef knife, serrated

Blender (regular or handheld) for shakes and smoothies

Corning® casserole heat and store dishes (great for heating frozen veggies)

Pyrex® glass bowls (good for mixing oatmeal, frittatas, eggs, pancakes)

Pepper grinder/mill

Assorted sizes of non-stick cookware, pans, pots
Colander, grater, spatulas, turners, tongs, large spoons, forks, and cooking utensils
Electronic timer
Cuisinart™ food processor
Kitchen-Aid™ stand mixer or handheld mixer
Assorted sizes of Tupperware™
Ziploc™ freezer bags, assorted sizes

Tip #47: Navigating the supermarket skillfully!

Supermarkets can be dangerous places for healthy eaters if you aren't prepared. The modern supermarket is cleverly designed to tempt shoppers into buying the products they really don't need. Store managers are creative, and you find yourself immediately confronted with high calories goodies that will shrink your wallet and expand your waist.

The first things that you see at the newest stores are baked goods and take-home prepared foods. We all know the obvious temptations of a bakery, but harder to resist are the sights of all that gorgeous take-out food, entrees, salads, sandwiches, wraps, side dishes, cheeses, olives, and appetizers – the hidden and real culprits to many of my clients' eating problems. Many of these foods look healthy but they have hidden fats and high calorie ingredients. The middle aisles of most stores are also danger areas and you need to be careful. Avoid the aisles specializing in cookies, crackers, snack foods, sugar soda, candy, junk foods, canned fruit, and commercial bread. Be weary of the "big bargain" and "healthy food" sections with their high calorie, fruit-sweetened cookies and cereals that are no better for your waist and heart than the regular versions.

The perimeter and far corners of the market is where you will often find the best and healthiest foods. The dairy, meat, fish, produce, and frozen vegetables are usually on the perimeter or the sections furthest away from the entrance. There are a few exceptions, I realize. I know first-hand as I used to manage a supermarket for a living. The cereal aisle has oatmeal, wheat germ, all bran, and shredded wheat, while the canned section contains tuna, salmon, tomato sauce, beans, vegetables, soups, and fat-free chili. The baking and spice aisle is good for trying new and interesting spices to liven up your food. There are also sugar-free sweeteners, low-sugar jams, sugar-free syrups, and sugar-free hot chocolate. Don't forget the condiment aisle with a multitude of choices for mustards, ketchups, salad dressings (fat-free), vinegars, salsa, and fat-free mayonnaise. If you must venture into the snack food aisle, buy non-fat microwave popcorn, fat-free potato chips, and baked taco or tortilla chips. Buy small portion-control sizes of fat-free pretzels and look for non/fat-free soy chips and root veggie chips.

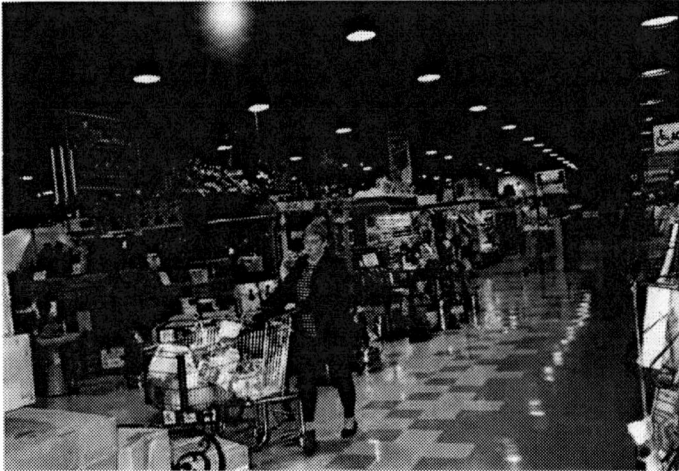

The latest innovation at the supermarket are the dinners-to-go, prepared meals, salad bars, and reheatable full dinners that require little or no preparation time for busy on-the-go people. The convenience and versatility of this concept is fantastic but making a healthy choice is the tricky part. Always go for the salad bar first and choose fresh vegetables, leafy greens, and fat-free dressing. Avoid croutons, mayo-based salads, and pudding desserts.

At the prepared foods case, some great choices include roast chicken or plain, grilled chicken breast. Plus, you might want to try any type of grilled meat, seafood or poultry. Use your own condiments from home to enliven these foods (salsas, mustards, salad dressings, etc.) Go for the vegetables, and the plain baked potatoes or sweet potatoes. Beans and lentil dishes are also good high-fiber choices, as are salads made with whole grains like barley, kashi, quinoa, or wheat berries. Ask the counter person to assist you when making low-fat food choices. They can be a good resource. The prepared food service is good for those who hate to cook and find themselves ordering Chinese or pizza for dinner. The only drawback is the expense, which is usually high and the frequency of visits to buy food every 2-3 days or more.

Tip #48: For the non-cook: become a "meal assembler"

Another great alternative to cooking is to be a *Heater-upper* or *microwave chef*. Using mostly frozen and convenience foods, you can create meals in minutes on a much lower budget. Many of my clients are on the "Lean Cuisine" program. This is a good portion-controlled meal that provides a satisfying and nutritious dining experience if eaten along with a big pre-packaged salad or a bowl of vegetables and low-calorie dessert. The choices among frozen entrees are incredibly vast and full of variety to suit any taste. Lean Cuisine™, Weight Watchers™, Healthy Choice™, and smaller regional brands offer hundreds of entrees and side dishes featuring foods you thought would be forbidden on most weight loss programs (e.g., spaghetti and meatballs, macaroni and cheese, enchiladas, Chinese stir-fry, beef stews, and even desserts, etc.).

As I've said before, the secret to success in using frozen entrees is PORTION CONTROL. It's not necessarily the type of food eaten. Remember there are no forbidden foods, ONLY FORBIDDEN WAYS TO EAT THEM. Yes, you can have macaroni and cheese, but you have to limit your serving size. You cannot eat a half a casserole and expect to lose weight. The secret is not WHAT, but HOW much. This is also the secret to lifelong success and getting off the "Diet Mentality" of ALL-OR-NOTHING thinking with regard to eating. This is why the "Lean Cuisine Program" works for many of my formerly overweight clients. Include all foods, even your favorite high fat treats, and you'll eventually learn to stop bingeing and either being "on" or "off" your diet.

Deprivation of your favorite food sets you up for bingeing later on, so eat small portions of your high fat, high-sugar treats (or limit the time and day you'll enjoy them). Eat moderate amounts of higher fat meats, starches, cereals, breads, and pastas and eat large amounts of vegetables, leafy greens, fresh fruit, and very lean protein (fish, turkey, buffalo, shellfish, non-fat dairy, eggs, cheese, and soy products.

Tip #49: Be a careful label reader!

The practice of deceptive labeling is one of my pet peeves. Most manufacturers know that most people don't usually read labels carefully on the foods we buy. It takes time most of us don't have during a shopping trip to be really careful with our choices by scrutinizing the labels. The most overlooked part of many items, especially individually- portioned snack food and low-fat baked goods is the serving size.

A good example (well, actually a bad example) is the fat-free muffin. If you need a breakfast muffin and have no other choice like yogurt, cottage cheese or a protein drink, then going fat-free is what I call a *better bad choice*. You go to the muffin aisle and look at the label and let's say that you see that the calorie count is 220 and the fat grams 0. Great! Not a bad way to go, you think. But wait – did you forget to check the servings per package? Of course, most of us do. The portions per package in this muffin total 2.5! Now, you realize this little low calorie treat is a whopper-sized 550 calories!

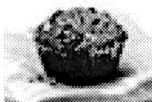

Another good example (or once again, a bad example) is the "healthy fruit juices" sold under the guise of low calorie health food. Nantucket Nectars™ labels their 12 ounce bottles as having 200 calories, but the portion is for only *half* the bottle. Their juice bottle contains a small, high-carb meal (400 calories) with three times the calories of a twelve ounce can of regular Coke™.

Deceptive labeling is especially prevalent in the health foods sections of most supermarkets. Cereals, cookies, candy, and baked goods are deemed virtuous by the "SUGAR FREE" label. Sugar-free does not mean it is free of sugar-based carbohydrates. It just means it has no white cane sugar and is sweetened with fructose, fruit juice, corn syrup, maltose, dextrose, raw cane juice, brown sugar, honey, molasses, or sorghum. Many of these products have higher calories than their regular counterparts. The truly sugar-free products are made with NutraSweet™, Splenda™, or Sweet & Low™ and will say it right on the label. Remember, all sugar, regardless of its origin, turns into glucose in the body (except the sugar substitutes) and too much will encourage fat storage. My advice is to avoid these "healthy" high-calorie foods, eat everything in its most natural state (fruit, veggies, natural protein), and enjoy the real treats you crave on a controlled basis once in a while. Remember the Caveman diet suggestions? You'll save a lot of money, be at your ideal weight, and feel happier overall.

Tip #50: Bargains are no bargain when it comes to calories!

It's stupefying and one of the great paradoxes of American life: often, it is easier and much cheaper to eat an unhealthy, high-sugar, and fat-laden diet. The major store bargains are usually the things we should avoid. Most products containing sugar, flour, and fat are easy to buy at rock-bottom prices. Major manufacturers are always making deals with supermarkets to feature these items in exchange for better prices. End displays are always loaded with potato chips, cookies, and sugary cereals. The healthiest foods are not usually on sale. Quality fresh produce, fish and shellfish, meats, and poultry are usually pricier if you buy the best quality and the leanest cuts. New stores like Fresh Fields®, Whole Foods®, and Trader Joes® along with other established national chains including Albertsons®, Winn-Dixie®, Stop & Shop®, and Kash N' Karry® have made healthy shopping a more enjoyable experience. Unfortunately, these supermarkets are more expensive; although they do offer more variety than most convenience and major food chain stores.

Farmers and ethnic markets offer a chance to get the freshest and best produce for a much lower price. If you live in a major metropolitan area or an area with an immigrant or ethnic population, you are likely to have Chinese or Asian markets, Middle Eastern, Indian, Spanish, Mexican, Italian, Russian, or European stores that offer possibly new and definitely interesting choices in low-fat foods, produce dairy products and meats.

Tip #51: Form a co-op group

Wholesale places like BJ's Price Club® and Sam's® are good for bargain hunters but you must be extra careful and shop not for what's cheap, but what will support your new healthy eating and lifestyle habits. This is a great opportunity to shop with a friend or group to split the cost and make quantities more manageable. Some of my clients have formed co-op shopping groups and shop together at major wholesalers, farmers markets, and ethnic markets. They have a chance to bond with each other and support one another in their weight-loss efforts. They also love to talk, swap recipe ideas, and share gym gossip. It's a fun outing for everyone that serves a useful purpose.

Co-op groups support each other in their struggles with food and exercise. This is also a great weekly social event that has for them become more of a weekly "supper club." It's fun and makes the whole idea of eating healthy more appealing. It also keeps them accountable to one another when I can't be there to support them. Each week one person takes a turn at assigning the types of food each person will make (meat, vegetables, chicken, fish, side dishes, snacks, and even desserts!). Supper clubs have a positive effect on the lives of those who try it because it gives them the support and encouragement of others also on the same path. TRY IT!

Another one of my clients, Rob, came up with a super idea. He went to a local culinary school and asked to post a notice on the bulletin board. The message read: In-home chef needed for part-time work. He was swamped with calls from eager young chef apprentices who wanted to make some extra cash and create foods that were tasty and healthy. He made suggestions on recipes and the calorie range he wanted, what types of food he was trying to avoid, and offered his library of low-fat cookbooks and back issues of *Cooking Light*. He was able to eat more consistently and healthfully even when his demanding career kept him at the office for 12 to 14 hours a day.

Tip #52: Hire a shopping pro

Finally, if you truly are too busy to shop and find it impossible to fit it into your schedule, consider hiring a pro to do it for you. Many trainers, including myself, are providing this as an additional service to clients to help them adhere to their program. Some people hire high school or college kids to the job. My Mom does some of my essentials shopping during my busy weeks. Do what ever it takes to get the job done. Don't let a lack of time be an excuse for failing on your eating program. Use the delivery service that some of the smaller markets provide. Surf the Internet to have things delivered to your door. Another great way to go is the weekly food delivery service from an Internet company called Diets to Go (http://www.DIETSTOGO.com) This is just one of the many locally and nationally-based services that provide busy people with healthy meals.

You can do it. It can be done. Start TODAY!

Tip #53: Cook at your own comfort level

Now that you've done your food shopping, it's time to unpack your booty and begin cooking those healthy, fat-reducing muscle-building meals. One of the first things you must do is to determine your level of competency and comfort in the kitchen. Ask yourself these questions in this **Cooking Comfort Level Quiz**. *Are you a . . .*

1. *"Foodie"* individual? In other words, are you a creative food person who enjoys food and cooking as a recreational hobby? Do you lust after the Williams & Sonoma™ catalog and dream of the day you'll install a dream kitchen with professional grade appliances? You will be much more successful in the long run because you control the type of food and the portions. You might also subscribe to *Cooking Light* magazine.

2. *"Heat and Cook"* type? Do you gravitate to simple, easy reheatable foods? Do you enjoy eating the same 15 foods over and over because they satisfy you without going to a lot of trouble? Enjoy pre-packaged, microwave dishes? Do you make instant mashed potatoes and oatmeal? Then you are a "Reheat Chef" and like to eat at home, but are not willing to spend a lot of time with extensive food preparation. Time is usually the issue with you, so you need to eat well and do it quickly without forethought. You will do well by following the easy assemble and eat recipes that require minutes of preparation but provide maximum nutrition.

3. *"Food Forgetter"* person? Are you someone who just FORGETS to eat? Are you consumed with your career or other goals and activities so that food is an afterthought? Do you look at food as something to give you energy and stop the rumbling in your stomach? Are you always ordering out, eating convenience food, or fast food because your home fridge is usually empty (except for leftover Chinese food containers) because you rarely

do supermarket shopping? IF SO, you need lots of support and must gradually change your relationship to food and eating. You need to have help in shopping, get the service of a personal chef, enlist your friends' help, and begin to make the lifestyle changes that will support your weight loss goals.

Whether you are a Creative Chef, Microwave Whiz, or a Takeout Tommy, you are always better off cooking and eating at home for several reasons.

<u>**Calorie and portion control**</u>. You know what you are putting in the dish as you can read the label on your frozen dinner and know exactly the calories, carbohydrates, and fat grams of your meal. You have to guess when you eat out.

<u>**Choices for healthy foods are much greater**</u>. Variety is what makes eating healthfully more fun and stimulating.

<u>**Fat control**</u>. Many of the seemingly healthy dishes at restaurants, take-out, and convenience food stores have hidden fats of which we're not aware. A healthy dish can be loaded with fat and excessive carbohydrates even if it's labeled low calorie, healthy, or lean.

The more you eat and prepare your meals at home, the more successful you'll be in the shortest time possible. Now that you realize the importance of cooking at home, you have four options to make it successful for you in the long run. By participating in the **Cooking Comfort Level Quiz**, you learned you have some choices based on your time, temperament, lifestyle, and budget. You can:

1. Cook yourself;
2. Use convenient heat and eat foods or "assembled meals";
3. Get healthy meals delivered from a company that specializes in diet and "clean food" lifestyle; or,
4. Hire a chef, apprentice, or local amateur cooking enthusiast part-time to cook and freeze your meals for you in your home.

Cooking for yourself is a wonderful experience if you have the time and the inclination. You may enjoy playing the role of chef or even aspire to cook professionally and eventually have your own show on a local or national cable TV food network! Or, you might be interested in hosting healthy dinner parties with your friends and family. You will do well, but you must be careful to maintain portion control and watch the HIGH-FAT components of your favorite recipes. Try the recipes in my book or use the recipes in the food magazines like *Cooking Light*. Buy the books of famous chefs and celebrities who have light and healthy cookbooks. The choice in cookbooks on healthy eating is overwhelming today. Also, there are local cooking demonstrations and classes that teach enlightened foods, healthy eating, and even videos on how to eat and enjoy the healthy lifestyle. Make this your hobby. Maybe you can help others who need assistance in cooking. Hey, it could be a new business for you and a way to express your creative food interest while maintaining a great body!

Using Convenience Foods is the Next Best Thing to Cooking from Scratch

As I mentioned before, you have an unprecedented number of choices to eat healthfully without going to a great deal of preparation. Supermarket take-out, local gourmet markets, ethnic cuisine, frozen dinners, pre-packaged, washed and cut salad greens and fresh vegetables, pre-cooked, ready-to-eat chicken and shrimp are just some of the ideas you can use to make delicious meals in minutes. Even 7-11® now carries low-fat cottage cheese, fruit yogurt, and Healthy Choice™ lunchmeat on whole wheat bread! There's never an excuse to order a pepperoni pizza (unless you really need it and are prepared to wear it or run a half marathon to burn it off).

Tip #54: Stick with basic recipes

The simplest way to create a habit of healthy cooking and eating is to find a small selection of favorite recipes and foods you enjoy and make them on a regular basis. As I've discussed previously, most people have a repertoire of about 15 basic food items they use over and over, so take advantage of this and don't make a big deal out of cooking. The Simpler, The Better. Many of my clients eat the same breakfast and lunch every day. They don't have to think and make decisions about food that interfere with their busy careers. The best time to make alternative choices is for meals at a restaurant on weekends or days off when life is less hectic and food can be enjoyed for pleasure and relaxation.

Use techniques that appeal to your tastes and time limitations. Some of my clients enjoy sautéing everything on the stove, while others like the longer, slower oven-baking process. The busy people, of course, use the microwave the most, some almost exclusively.

Read the food magazines that feature FAST & EASY dinners. Buy cookbooks featuring recipes ready in "Fifteen Minutes or Less," or with limited ingredients (Rosanne Gold has a series of cookbooks featuring three ingredients or less). CHOOSE 15 OF YOUR FAVORITE RECIPES AND USE THEM OVER AND OVER. If you are totally foreign and uncomfortable in the kitchen, go to an evening cooking class for a brief intro to healthy culinary techniques. Local community colleges, restaurant training schools, and healthy food supermarkets (including Fresh Fields®, Trader Joes®, and Wild Oats®, among others) sponsor chef seminars that will give you great ideas and inspiration.

If you've made up your mind that cooking will never be part of your lifestyle, consider having your food delivered by one of the online food services. Ediets® (http://www.ediets.com) and DietstoGo® (http://www.dietstogo.com) offer a food delivery service that is reasonable and low in calories. Order healthy choices off your favorite local restaurant menu and have it delivered. Or, order Chinese take-out, but take care and go with steamed veggies, soup, and absolutely nothing fried or in a sweet and sour sauce. Choose take-out with the same careful vigilance as if you were at a restaurant. Assume everything you're ordering has hidden fat and ask them to make it as fat free and light as possible. Even pizza can be ordered with light cheese, extra sauce, and grilled vegetables to save hundreds of waist-expanding calories.

Here's an example of one of my client's "**FAVORITE 15**" and his shopping list for two weeks.

1. Oatmeal with NutraSweet™, raisins, and cottage cheese topping
2. Puffed wheat cereal with sugar-free maple syrup
3. Non-fat grilled cheese sandwich and canned soup
4. Corn tortillas filled with scrambled egg beaters, non-fat cheese, and topped with hot salsa
5. Egg white omelette with vegetable filling, light whole wheat toast with no sugar jam and non-fat butter
6. White tuna in water with canned artichokes on a bed of pre-washed bag of salad with non-fat Caesar dressing
7. Frozen Italian vegetable combination microwaved with two tablespoons of parmesan cheese and butter substitute
8. Sliced apples with chunks of low-fat cheddar cheese
9. Cottage cheese topped with chopped dates
10. Fresh fruit salad mixed into non-fat vanilla yogurt
11. Weight Watchers™ or Healthy Choice™ frozen dinner entrees
12. Purdue™ Low-fat chicken cutlets topped with non-fat mozzarella and Hunts™ low-cal tomato sauce
13. Smoked salmon, chopped egg whites, capers, onions, and dill with non-fat sour cream
14. Jell-O™ sugar-free non-fat pudding mixed into MetRx™ protein drink or plain yogurt cups
15. Veggie, tuna, or salmon burger with ketchup and relish with homemade non-fat coleslaw and non-fat potato chips

Favorite snacks include:

1. Protein shakes
2. Popcorn
3. Sushi-to-go
4. Protein bars
5. Small, non-fat yogurt cups

Jim Hart, A.C.E.

Along with his two-week shopping list. . .

1 box, regular oatmeal
1 individual box, raisins
1 box, NutraSweet™ or Splenda™
1 bag, puffed wheat or rice
2 bottle, sugar-free maple syrup
3 containers, non-fat cottage cheese
2 packs, non-fat American cheese
1 loaf, 40 calorie/slice bread
3 cans, soup (vegetable, barley, chicken & rice)
1 jar, spicy Grey Poupon™ mustard
1 pack, corn tortillas
2 cartons, Egg Beaters™
3 dozen eggs
2 jars, chunky hot salsa jars
1 jar, Smuckers™ no-sugar jam
1 squeeze bottle, Smart Squeeze™ butter
3 bags, assorted frozen vegetables
3 cans, white tuna packed in water
2 cans, artichoke hearts
2 bags, Dole™ pre-washed salad
1 bottle, non-fat Caesar dressing
1 container, 8% parmesan grated cheese
4 Fuji apples
1 container, cheddar soy cheese
1 can, chopped fruit
2 containers, vanilla or plain non-fat yogurt
4 frozen dinners (Weight Watchers™ or Healthy Choice™)
1 pack, Purdue™ chicken cutlets
1 bag, non-fat mozzarella or provolone cheese
1 bottle, low-cal tomato sauce (Hunts™, Ragu™, or Healthy Choice™)
4 oz. smoked salmon
1 bottle, capers
1 container, non-fat sour cream
1 red onion
1 ounce, fresh dill

3 boxes, non-fat, sugar-free Jell-O™ pudding (butterscotch, white chocolate, pistachio)
1 box, Garden Burgers™
1 box, tuna burgers
1 bottle, ketchup
1 bottle, relish
1 bag, fresh pre-chopped cole slaw mix
1 bottle, non-fat Russian dressing
1 bag, Lays™ non-fat potato chips
1 dozen assorted low-cal yogurts

At the health food store or vitamin store . . .

12 assorted protein bars (under 6 g fat, under 30 g carbs, and greater than 20 g protein)
MetRx™ Vanilla shake mix
Whey Protein™ bars (chocolate)
Udo's Choice Fish Oil™ capsules
Multi-vitamins and mineral supplements
Glucosamine sulfate and chondraitin for joints
Glutamine for faster muscle growth
Vitamin C & E for immune-boosting and anti-oxidant protection

Tip #55: More mental & motivational shortcuts to success in sticking with your program

Arm yourself with motivational bullets and the armor of these gentle reminders to assure success for your immediate goals and for a future of health and fitness. THESE ARE THINGS THAT HAVE WORKED FOR ME AND HUNDREDS OF CLIENTS OVER MY LAST DECADE AS A PERSONAL TRAINER.

ASK YOURSELF, "Am I on a diet or am I committed to a lifestyle?"
There is a big distinction to draw between living a healthy lifestyle and being on a diet to lose a few pounds. How do you know you are finally living a healthy lifestyle and not on another "fitness kick" or fad diet binge? Here are some things you'll notice in your day-to-day thoughts and behaviors to know where you stand:

Scenario 1
You exercise because you enjoy it and like the way it makes you feel

Vs.

You punish yourself and exercise because you feel guilty about overeating. Extra treadmill time will wash away the sin of gluttony.

Scenario 2

You eat foods that give you pleasure and you enjoy in moderation and balance. You recognize that you have boundaries with certain foods in difficult situations

Vs.

You choose unappealing, plain monotonous "diet" foods that you feel you must eat in order to reach your goals.

Scenario 3

You recognize that some foods may not support your goals for a low-fat body, but you crave them. Rather than depriving yourself, you welcome the craving and ask, "Is there something that will satisfy me without the additional fat and calories?" You might find a substitute or eat ¼ to ½ of the food you desire.

Vs.

Your cravings are driving you crazy! You just don't have any will power. Once you start eating that food, you can't stop. You're just no good at dieting, so, why bother? If you can't do it 100%, you're not doing it at all. You are so undisciplined.

Scenario 4

You know some days your eating habits are a little less than ideal. In fact, some days, you're totally off the mark, but you're ready to pick up your good habits at the next meal and JUST EAT LIGHTLY and healthfully.

Vs.

You screwed up totally today. I might as well finish these cookies since I've blown it so badly. I'll start again on Monday. I might as well order that pepperoni pizza and just enjoy myself for now.

What Makes the Difference?

MINDFUL AWARENESS	*Vs.* MINDLESS CONSUMPTION
Giving into child-like impulses	*Vs.* Making adult-like choices
Recognizing wants are not always needs	*Vs.* Feeling deprived for not getting what you want

Remember the Rolling Stones song lyrics "You can't always get what you want. Sometimes, *you get what you need*?!"

When the going gets tough . . .

The real work in changing your life and your eating habits begins after the initial enthusiasm wears off. We all know how wonderful and rosy things are at the beginning of a relationship. We fall "head over heels" for a new partner. Next, we begin the courtship, the dating, and eventually plan the wedding, the honeymoon and our life together. But soon after the honeymoon, memories fade, and the reality of day to day living with another human being take hold. The foibles and faults of your beloved become more pronounced. You may sometimes wonder if you can spend the rest of your life with this person and you ask yourself, "What have I gotten myself into?" The realization is a wake-up call, a reminder that your relationship is a work in progress. It will take effort, compromise, patience, and courage to continue making it work day after day. The mature person recognizes the true nature of relationships – a system of getting our needs met through compromise, negotiation, sharing, giving, and being the best we can be. This is the same way you must approach your new commitment to eating healthy and exercise. Think of it as a relationship, from dating through honeymoon to the day to day sacrifices and compromises you must make to keep it alive and thriving. The rewards for sticking it out are wonderful and beyond measure!

The Splurge!

I've mentioned it before, but "taking a splurge" is truly amazing enough to reiterate time and again. The splurge is your chance to release your psychological pressure valve and let off steam. Each time you allow yourself a special treat you diminish its power and significance in your life. It's a good way to have long-term success in your eating and fitness program. It's OK to splurge on occasion. You can relax and enjoy the foods you crave:
- Go to a great restaurant and order what you like
- Buy the finest ingredients for a special dinner
- Get exactly the thing you've been craving on this one special day, drive out of your way if necessary
- Have a guilt-free celebration with friends on your birthday or special occasion

Tip #56: Practice the six rituals.

Having a daily, habitual system will reinforce your commitment to maintaining the eating and exercise habit.

#1 KEEP A JOURNAL

- Keep a journal of your daily food consumption and log of your workouts (writing it makes you accountable and gives you an objective view.
- Review in your journal the situations, people, places, and things that cause problems
- Ask what is holding you back and how you could move ahead. What or who do you need to help you get there (i.e. a workout partner or less restaurant meals, etc.)?
- Be thankful and grateful for the accomplishments you've made so far and don't beat yourself up for not being perfect.
- Set new goals and dates for their achievement. Make sure these goals are in line with what you value most (low body fat %'s, better cardio capacity, more energy, better performance for sport, bigger muscles, etc.).
- Write daily affirmations that help you to move towards your goal.

Remember these from before? They're worth repeating here!

Sample Affirmations:
1. "I'm doing everything I need to do today to reach my goal of 10% body fat."
2. "I eat only those foods that give me energy and keep me lean and low fat."
3. "I'm making good choices today that support my physical goals."
4. "I spend a little extra time today planning and cooking the meals that help me move towards washboard abs."

5. "I make compromises and sacrifices today that give me the time I deserve for my weight training and cardio program."

2 READ POSITIVE INSPIRATION

Set your tone for the day. Read motivational, inspirational, and supportive books, articles, or websites first thing in the morning. Doing the reading will help you become better physically, emotionally, spiritually, mentally, or will help advance your career and relationships with others. The reading or meditating can come in the form of self-help, religious, philosophical, psychology, Buddhist wisdom, or something from the Bible or Book of Tao.

Whatever you do, stay away from watching TV and reading newspapers, useless magazines, or radio talk shows first thing in the morning. These things, while useful for many other purposes, are candy for the mind that is trying to start new habits. Start your day by reading something positive, uplifting, and worthwhile. The inspirational reading is protein for the mind; it stays with you longer, satisfies, and helps you to grow (literally and figuratively).

#3 EXERCISE EARLY IN YOUR DAY

Exercise first thing in the MORNING. If you want to truly make a commitment to a healthy lifestyle, the best time to exercise is early in your day. There are less distractions, you are focused, and clear. The body responds better and you burn more calories all throughout the day because you have super-charged your metabolism. When my clients put exercise first, they surprisingly find that crises, emergencies, and work-related deadlines don't get in the way — unlike when they reserve their exercise for late in the day.

Doing it first says you have made it *Priority #1* in your life and it comes before anything else. You make a powerful statement to yourself and it sets you above all others who talk about working out, but don't adhere to their promises. You put "your money where your mouth is" when you train in the morning. As a trainer, I notice the gym members who come in consistently year after year are "the early morning exercisers."

#4 LEARN FROM OTHERS

Find out what other people have done to maintain long-term, successful weight loss and how they have built head-turning physiques. <u>Don't try to go at it alone</u>. Find someone you have noticed who has made a profound physical change and ask them what worked and what didn't. Don't be afraid. Most people are flattered and will gladly share their thoughts with you. Read diet and exercise books written by either experts who have great success with long-term weight loss or those who have lost weight and maintained their new habits for at least five years or more.

#5 WRITE A PRESUME!!

Here's another point mentioned previously that I believe deserves more attention. What is a presume? It's a plan with goal dates that presumes what you'll be doing with your future – a future made by your choices. One of my clients wrote a timeline into the next five years about the people, places, and things that were instrumental in helping him to slowly and gradually lose weight and keep up his exercise habit. Here is an excerpt from his journal dated January 5, 2004 (remember, he's projecting into the future):

> Well, I made it through a tough holiday season, but this year I didn't allow my usual impulses to eat take over. At the Christmas parties, with the huge buffets, I simply ate some oatmeal before the party to calm down my hunger. I followed the "Rule of ½" and just ate half portions of the foods I was really craving. I skipped the starchy potato and rice dishes in favor of a double vegetable portion and avoided the rolls so I could allot my calories to ½ portions of the desserts I was really craving. Last year, I would have hovered around the buffet (I eat when I'm nervous and in unfamiliar social situations). Instead, I set a goal of introducing myself to three people I didn't know and having a conversation. I did not allow myself to eat until I reached this goal, and it really works! This hasn't been a perfect time for my eating. I've managed to only lose about 1 pound over Christmas and New Year's, but compared to last year, when I gained 10 pounds, I'm doing so much better and I feel good myself. I even met and have been dating one of the guests I introduced myself to at the Christmas party!

Writing a presume helps to put your subconscious to work for you. It's effortless and easy. Write a scenario that you would like to see happen, add dates, times, places, and people and watch what happens. Reread once a week to reinforce and you will start to see gradual changes that turn into realized goals, accomplishments, and achievements! Things will happen that you had previously thought were impossible. A presume is another thing you can write and review in your morning quiet time.

#6 USE POST-IT or MEDICINE CHEST MOTIVATION

One of my special tricks I use is to reinforce my goals through hanging Post-it reminders at places where I will see them during my daily rituals. I post notes inside my bathroom cabinet, at work inside my locker, both inside **and** on the refrigerator, on the dashboard, and on the bedroom mirror. These little helpers maintain my commitment and reinforce my goals and habits through repetition. Some of my mantras or Post-its include:

- I eat what I need to maintain washboard abs and muscular definition.
- I think about the choices I make today. Do they help or hinder me?
- I do everything I need to do to be healthy, happy, joyful, and at peace.
- I always have better choices for myself.

Tip #57: Fifteen golden rules of wisdom

1. Create small wins/victories for yourself

The subconscious mind has the final say about how you feel about the range of your success or failure. Your mind is like a computer that sees everything black or white – that's why it's important to start out slow with small baby steps. A goal of five minutes done every day is consistently better than a goal of 30 minutes consistently missed. You will benefit from setting small, reachable goals first and **DO IT DAILY**. This is how you build the exercise habit into your life and become more successful.

2. Be a rebel

Go against the tide of typical American thinking. Don't believe the advertising, diet gurus, infomercials, and all the "lose weight quick" schemes. Act as if you have found "IT!" Remember those bumper stickers from the Seventies – "*I FOUND IT!*"? Act as if you have a big secret, as if every other diet, exercise, and weight loss plan that your co-workers, brother-in-law and most of North America is on is just old hat, or so "LY" (Last Year) as they say in the fashion industry. When people ask you for your secret, tell them your BIG secret is a moderate diet that includes all foods and a consistent lifestyle of exercise and fun!

3. Get Real – The rule of 21

Wake up and smell the coffee! Acknowledge to yourself and others how difficult and life-changing the process of diet and exercise is. Ironically, by realizing the fact it's going to be tough, it prepares you to do better with the gremlins that keep you from success. It will take twenty-one days to break the old habit and twenty-one days to reinforce the new habits. Mentally preparing yourself for this from the beginning cuts away all the illusions of grandeur and high expectations of immediate gratification. If you can change and maintain a habit for 42 days, you can keep it for the rest of your life. Ask yourself, "Am I ready to make that commitment?"

4. It's 90% Mental!

Remember that exercise and eating habits are 90% mental gymnastics. Most of our resistance to eating right and exercising comes from our mental dialogue and the things we tell ourselves. The ever-present mental chatter in our head is the thing that creates the problem with sticking to a program. Volumes have been written on this subject and the bottom line is . . . Your excuses for not exercising are NOT PHYSICALLY BASED 90% of the time (unless you are an advanced athlete or over- trained bodybuilder). Your body can handle whatever you give it. It is the mind that holds us back and stops our progress and not our physical bodies.

5. Don't drive yourself crazy over counting calories.

If you've been unsuccessful at following the calorie formulas, keep it simple by following my Caveman eating guidelines. You know it from the previous chapters in the book, but here it is in a nutshell: STRIVE TO EAT EVERYTHING IN ITS MOST NATURAL AND UNPROCESSED STATE 80% of the time!

6. You don't need your wants

Numerous studies have proven that CRAVINGS and obsessions on a particular type of food have not any rational or physical basis. They are purely psychological and based on cues from our environment. Past conditioning and our PAST BEHAVIOR regarding certain foods become habits when we encounter situations, people, places, and emotions that have food as reward or punishment attached to them.

Do you remember being rewarded with dessert when you were "good" or were you soothed with a lollipop when you fell and scraped a knee? Does a trip to the seaside boardwalk or lakeside swimming beach bring back memories of pizza, caramel corn, fudge, and cotton candy that you devoured as a teenager? THESE ARE EXAMPLES OF TRIGGERS THAT CAUSE "CRAVINGS."

Of course we **want** these foods because they taste good and they make us temporarily feel good, but you don't **need** pizza to survive. You do need a variety of good lean protein, fruits, and vegetables to survive and thrive in a healthy, energetic state. Keep this is mind when a craving hits you and realize you can make a better choice. Don't be afraid of a paper tiger. FACE

THE CRAVING AS A WAVE AT THE BEACH THAT WILL APPROACH, WASH OVER YOU, AND SUBSIDE!

7. Twins of Diet Damage Control: the *"better bad choices"* and the *"rule of half"*

Better Bad Choices: Like most Americans, we always find ourselves in compromising situations that make it difficult to stay with our eating plan. Most people don't eat right because it's close to impossible in Twenty-first century America. We've got our fast food, junk snacks, and huge portions at both upscale and downscale restaurants. When faced with a buffet of fattening foods (e.g., a heavy restaurant meal or fast food dish), I recommend ordering items with the lowest calories and the smallest sizes. Refer to the tips I give you earlier on eating out and making good choices. If you eat at McDonald's®, go with the chicken breast sandwich over the Big Mac™ and save 400 calories. At vending machines, stay away from Snickers™ bars and have a bag of pretzels and save about 200 calories or more. When everyone is going out for ice cream, have a dish of frozen yogurt instead and save up to 500 calories.

The Rule of Half. **IF** you must eat the real thing, <u>just eat half</u>. Share the other half, or throw it out. When you give into cravings, it's usually for high fat, high sugar foods. A half portion of pecan pie is 325 calories. A half bag of French Fries is about 200 calories. A half portion of chocolate mousse is 250 calories. You can derive great satisfaction from eating the real thing in small amounts while still staying on track with your healthy habits. So don't deprive yourself. Once in a while, it's good to eat what you really want, but stay within limits by following the "Twins of Damage Control."

8. Finding time to exercise is a myth

As I mentioned earlier, there is no such thing as "finding time to exercise and eat right." In our busy, hectic lifestyles, no one has "spare time" to exercise. It's like spare money. You can choose to budget your money and time, but none of it is EXTRA, none of it is spare.

We all have the same 24 hours, no more, no less. So, forget about "finding time" and let's talk about developing a way to budget your time to slowly develop the successful, consistent habits that help you create the body you want. Time management is not about time but about habit development. It's taking something that you're not used to doing (EXERCISE AND EATING

Jim Hart, A.C.E.

RIGHT) and TURNING IT INTO SOMETHING YOU'RE NOT USED TO DOING WITHOUT!

How do you develop a habit? Take small, gradual, and consistent steps over time. Think of a baby as it begins the process of being crib-bound to running around the house. The baby starts with a slow crawl, then a faster crawl, a crawl up the steps, then standing while holding onto the couch. Next, the baby walks while holding onto the coffee table. And finally one day he learns to stand upright on his own and takes a few solo steps and begins walking. Soon, the baby is zipping around the house, eluding his exhausted parents.

Let's consider another scenario . . .. What if the baby, while only able to lie in the crib, decided to get up and run around the house? Without any intermediate steps and goals, after a few tries and numerous slips and falls, the baby would give up in discouragement and decide not to do it again because he thinks he really sucks at running. Phew! I'm tired just thinking about making such a leap!

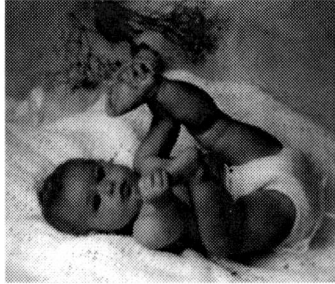

Well, isn't that what most people do with exercise goals? One might say, "I'm starting a new program this week – 45 minutes of cardio and three days of strength training." Wrong idea if you are just starting out. Most people who set immediate, high expectations soon find they've bit off more than they could possibly handle, give it up and blame it on a lack of time. Set up the habit so you can win. Do small 5 – 10-minute increments consistently for three weeks and see if it doesn't make you feel victorious and proud of yourself.

9. There's no such thing as will power . . . all that counts is your action in the present moment.

I've borrowed this from Zen Buddhism. It is deceptively simple but profoundly powerful and it works if you practice it. When faced with an overwhelming task (losing 25 pounds, running a marathon, getting a college degree), we tend to get bogged down by looking at the big picture. Many people obsess about the time it will take to lose the weight, the hundreds of miles to train before the race, and the countless hours of studying and expense of attending four years of college.

To be successful, you must take it in small bites and break it down into day by day tasks. Moment to moment decisions and choices will move you towards your goal. Each action you take (deciding to have fruit today instead of cookies) leads you toward the desired goal; losing one pound at a time. In running you take one step at a time (you've heard the phrase "the journey of a thousand miles begins with a single step"), and complete one mile at a time. In college you take one class at a time, read one chapter at a time, and complete one semester at a time.

Life is a series of moments where you are given choices to move <u>towards</u> or <u>away</u> from the goal you've CHOSEN. No matter how badly you screw up, there's always another moment waiting for you to make a choice or take a good action. Only your action in the present is what counts. The past is gone, the future doesn't exist, relieve yourself of the burden of trying to control the future or correct the past and <u>be here now</u>. For more on staying in the present read Eckhart Tolle's book, <u>The Power of Now</u>.

10. Allow yourself a cheat day

I can't stress enough the importance of allowing yourself "to let your hair down," release (or at least loosen) your grip in the reins of strict dieting and just eat whatever strikes your fancy. You can do it for a single restaurant meal, a weekend day, or designate one to two special occasions during the course of a week where you will consciously eat and enjoy whatever you want.

Being strict all the time will lead to binges and yo-yo dieting extremes. Remember it takes several days for your body to add weight. In most cases it creeps up slowly, because your body does not want to make metabolic changes too quickly. A few large and indulgent meals once or twice a week can make you feel better emotionally, physically, and mentally.

11. Don't listen to the voice that wants to quit

For many years I have been able to do my morning runs on those "off days." When I just didn't feel motivated I told myself:

I will only run for a short 10 minutes – if
I still feel lousy, I will turn back and call it a day.

Guess what? 95% of the time, I keep on running. Your body takes time to adjust to the metabolic and physical demands you place on it during the first stages of aerobic exercise the body, will protest loud and clear it's displeasure with this new workload you're asking it to do. TOUGH IT OUT! Keep telling yourself it will get easier and more enjoyable in 10-15 minutes. Do whatever it takes, don't quit, and think how good aerobic exercise makes you look and how good you feel after a workout.

12. The $10,000,000.00 Question

How fast would you run if someone offered you this sum of money if you could run five miles, six days a week for six months? Would that motivate you? What excuses would you use? Would you think twice about prioritizing this in your daily To Do list?

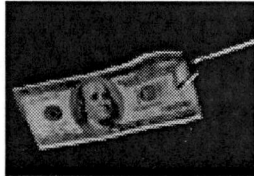

How much mental, emotional, and physical energy would you put into daily exercise, sleep habits, healthy eating for immune-boosting, optimum performance to prevent sick days? I guarantee you'd be performing and looking like an Olympic athlete within six months. Why? Because your heightened motivation magically removed the roadblocks and problems that that held you back in the past. THINK ABOUT IT. WHAT WOULD YOU BE DOING RIGHT NOW IF YOU WERE IN THE FIFTH MONTH OF YOUR QUEST FOR TEN MILLION DOLLARS? What would your daily schedule look like? What would you be eating, drinking, and doing to keep your body in top shape?

13. Think like a Catholic, trained athlete, military recruit, or firefighter trainee

With few exceptions, many of the most successful people I train are practicing Catholics (or former Catholics sometimes called Recovering Catholics), previously trained athletes, military men, or firefighters. Why? I only have anecdotal evidence and it's surely based on observation but it's because they are brought up in a religion, industry, or discipline complete with rules, regulations, and minimum standard requirements. To remain in the Catholic faith, for example, I am required to attend a certain number of masses, practice the Ten Commandments, and refrain from certain behaviors and sins that unless confessed will cost me an eternity in the fires of hell. Now that's motivation! Catholics are basically given a clear-cut formula for salvation. You are told what to do, when to do it, and what will happen if you don't. There's no questioning, no room for interpretation, no exceptions – it's all black and white.

Now, if you apply the same way of thinking to diet and exercise, it becomes easy to eat right, exercise consistently, lose fat and build muscle. The clients who follow my instructions for eating, aerobics, and strength training without fail are successful, happier, and look better than those who bend or break the rules. Sometimes it's easier if you don't have to decide. It's less mental work to just do what you're told without question. Try it for a week. It will be hard but when it gets tough "offer it up" and your suffering will help free the souls in purgatory.

14. Use tools, gadgets, and toys

To add fun and variety to your workout, consider using some of the many products that monitor, motivate, and measure your progress. Heart rate monitors, motion detecting distance counters, pedometers, and calorie trackers can add an element of challenge. Heart rate monitors are incredibly useful tools that assist to reach the fat-burning calorie range with more accuracy and precision. Knowing your heart rate while you run will help you to burn more calories more efficiently and in less time. Motion detectors and pedometers tell you exactly how far you walk or run, while the calorie trackers will give you an objective picture of how many calories you really burn during your normal working hours.

As a trainer, I require all my clients to use a Cal Trac™ calorie tracker for two weeks and to use a heart rate monitor at the beginning of their

Jim Hart, A.C.E.

cardio programs. It's a real eye-opener for most people when they find out how many calories they actually burn during the day (the number is usually much less than they originally thought). Using the Cal Trac™ and the heart rate monitor shows how they are sometimes going either too slow or too fast to effectively burn fat. I recommend a base model Polar™ heart rate monitor in addition to the Cal Trac™. Sporting goods stores carry these products or you can consult their webpages.

15. Rise Above Your Plateau

Getting stuck or stale in your workout progress, weight loss, or strength goals is a common problem for people pursuing fitness goals.

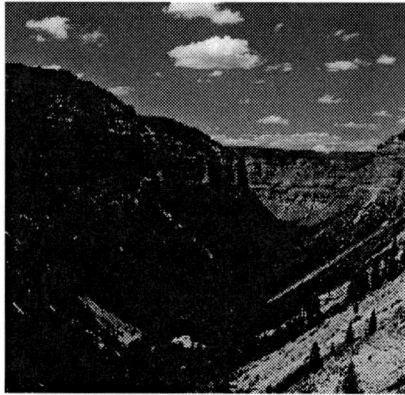

After the initial first months, progress naturally slows as the body adapts to the new routine and eating regimen. Here are ways to get off the plateau and start moving ahead:

IN WEIGHT TRAINING

Change your workout often with:

Supersets (doing two or three exercises consecutively with NO REST)
Super-slow lifting (each repetition takes approximately 10 seconds)
Circuit training
All dumbbell training
Raising and lowering weights

Increasing reps, changing repetitions, raising speed of reps
Decreasing rest periods/alternating rest periods
Change the order of body parts
Try a new gym
Run through routine backwards
Add push-ups, dips, chin-ups
Get a partner or HIRE A TRAINER TO DO IT WITH YOU!

IN CARDIOVASCULAR AEROBIC EXERCISE

Change your workout often by:

Trying new classes
Testing new machines
Run faster for shorter distances and vice versa
Take up a new sport – join a team
Try a different time of day to train
Run or walk a new route
Use gadgets and monitors
Get a partner or hire a coach
Train for an event

JUMP HIGHER THAN YOUR PLATEAUS IN EATING WELL:

Consider these options each for one week:

Try three new fruits or vegetables
Add 35 grams of fiber a day to your diet
Eat ¼ less portion than you normally consume
(Conversely, if trying to gain, raise portions ¼)
Eliminate one type of junk food from your diet
Give up alcohol and drinks with sugars or syrups
Avoid flour-based products
Try a new restaurant and test your healthy ordering skills
When tempted, carry an optional healthy alternative on your person
Drink six to eight large glasses of water/day
Practice "mindful awareness" (eat w/o reading, watching TV, or doing anything else)

Journal the problematic people, places, situations, and things that make you overeat

Keep a food journal

Tip #58: How to deal with emotional or stress-related eating

An interesting and unexplained paradox is that stress makes some people want to eat more. *The New York Times* reported an unusual side effect from the September 11 tragedy. As a way to cope with the stress and aftermath of the unsettling events, New Yorkers began eating more home-style meals, comfort, and junk foods (*New York Times*, October 23, 2001) Scientists and eating disorder experts can't agree on why this happens, but the problem remains – stressful situations are sometimes a major issue for people trying to lose weight.

When I discuss weight loss with my clients, the issue of stress arises repeatedly. Some people point to a specific stressful event to explain why they gained weight in the first place. Others say stress makes them want to eat and "nibble and nosh" all day long. While others maintain that stress from job, family, or the environment threatens their efforts and puts them at risk for a relapse into their old ways of overeating.

If you feel stress if influencing your eating, ask yourself some questions:

1. When you feel pressure to accomplish something, do you feel pulled towards food, and start thinking about eating?
2. If you were sitting at a desk working on a deadline, would you want to be nibbling?
3. Do you use food to make you feel better when you are stressed?
4. Does stress, sadness, emotional upset, depression, "bad hair days," influence you eat more?

If you answered yes to any of these questions, then stress and eating are linked for you in some very important ways. The question is what to do about it. **There are two solutions. The first is to respond to stress with other activities aside from eating. Below, are suggestions of activities**

incompatible with eating and these ideas will distract you from bad eating behaviors:

     Surf the Internet
     Call a friend
     Take a shower or bubble bath
     Go to a movie
     Take a short walk or a longer country walk
     Go for a drive
     Have sex – or read a sexy book
     Read a favorite magazine
     Go to the gym for a ½ hour
     Ride your bike
     Work in your garden or buy new flowers
     Wash your car
     Buy someone a gift
     Work on your hobby
     Volunteer – or do something nice for someone
     Visualize your ideal body

Make up five to 10 of your own right here:

1.

2.

3.

4.

5.

6.

7.

8.

9.

10.

Make them fun, doable, and enjoyable at a moment's notice. Things you can spring into action quickly when the overeating urges hit work best. If you distract yourself for even just a few minutes, the urge to eat will often pass. Studies show that hunger comes and goes during the day so by pausing and not impulsively reaching for food, it gives you time to think and ride out the temptation.

The second part of the solution is to reduce the stress in our life which will not only help you in managing your eating, but will affect all other areas of your life as well. I can't do a fully detailed discourse on stress management here (that's another book entirely), but I can give you some helpful tips that work for my clients. I recommend a wonderful book called Mastering Stress: A Lifestyle Approach, by Dr. David Barlow and Ronald Ropee. Also, consider books or learning to meditate and live a more "Zen-like' lifestyle. The Idiots Guide to Zen Living is a helpful introduction to meditating and putting peaceful, Eastern ideas into our hectic Western lifestyle.

I make two suggestions for dealing with stress in the moment. First, you can learn to use relaxation techniques. A simple, five-minute break while consciously focusing on your breath will usually break the stress cycle. Or, just take five deep breaths when the temptation to overeat begins. Second, I recommend that you learn appraisal techniques. When an event occurs in our lives we appraise the situation and then respond. The appraisal determines the response. One person who receives a poor evaluation from his boss might make a negative appraisal, suffer a blow to self-esteem, and feel depressed. Someone else may take a more positive appraisal. The optimist could view the criticism as constructive and sees a chance to improve work performance, get a better position, and ultimately a higher salary.

Learning relaxation, meditation, and better appraisal techniques can change your attitude about the stressful situations that are an inevitable part of life. You do have choices when dealing with things other than eating excessively. Don't put your body at risk for obesity, along with all the health-related problems you've work so hard to overcome.

THINK, CHOOSE, WIN!

Tip #59: How to prevent slip-ups

On the road to reaching your fitness goal, the bumpiest parts have to do with eating and dealing with temptations. Losing weight and maintaining a healthy shape is one of the greatest challenges you will ever face. Therefore, on a day-to-day basis, it is important to accept your mistakes, learn from them, and deal constructively with situations as they arise.

There are two paths to success. The first is to avoid or prevent mistakes and slip-ups. The second is to respond to slips with coping techniques that put you in control.

There are three levels of slip-ups:
1. A **LAPSE** is an occasional slight error that involves eating one piece of a high fat food or indulging at inappropriate times.
2. A **RELAPSE** occurs when lapses are strung together and you return to your former habits of overeating and poor food choices.
3. A **COLLAPSE** is when the relapse continues for a long period of several weeks or more. It's a negative downward trend with decreasing odds for reversal. Often, the person gives up and begins another yo-yo dieting cycle.

It is important to distinguish between a **LAPSE** from a **RELAPSE**. A single lapse does not mean you are falling off your program and into a relapse. You need to view a lapse as a temporary slip and respond positively to these inevitable setbacks. Identify your high-risk situations and list those situations that threaten your eating. Some examples include:
- Dining at a restaurant
- Feasting at Mom's home-cooked dinners
- Eating at a wedding
- Feelings of stress, anxiety, depression
- Indulging over the holidays, Halloween, Valentine's Day, Easter candy, etc.
- Walking near Burger King® or your favorite fast food restaurant
- Eating at a company party or picnic

List your greatest high-risk situations here:

1.

2.

3.

4.

5.

Once you've identified the situations you can plan ahead. Be sure to eat often and follow the Caveman rules as often as possible. Additionally, here are two great techniques that I ask my clients to use:

*1. **Outlast the urge*** – Remember that an urge disappears sometimes if you just wait it out! Easier said than done, I know, but think of how good and powerful you feel when you succeed!

*2. **Use the WAVE ANALOGY***. Eating urges are like waves. They begin small, crest, break, then subside and fade away. The wave analogy is much different than the way most of us think about urges. We feel the wave building and getting stronger and the only way out is to eat. But, by eating we only reinforce this habit and make the wave stronger and more frequent. If you can let the urge go, by waiting it out, it will weaken and fade into obscurity.

Pretend that you're surfing (on the north shore of Hawai'i) as the wave rolls in you can battle it and be wiped out or you can maintain your balance and ride the wave until it subsides. Being a good "URGE SURFER" involves identifying the bad food urges early in their development and then readying your skills to ride the wave. If a wave is upon you full strength before you recognize it, you'll wipe out.

Sometimes you need more than just waiting it out, so try using the "alternative activities and techniques that are incompatible with eating (see TIP #58)". When you get the urge, DO SOMETHING ELSE. If you use bad food urges as a signal for positive activity, eating will become less rewarding and the old associations between urges and eating will diminish.

Jim Hart, A.C.E.

Remember, some eating habits have nothing to do with hunger. They're merely mental or emotionally stimulated associations that cue your urges. You can learn to make new associations with food and be successful and conquer those urges. For example, each time you have a bad food hunger urge begin surfing the computer or consider a visit to an Ediets chat room (see http://www.ediets.com) and get support from others struggling with the same situation. Consider a great self-hypnosis course that several of my clients have used successfully called "The Smart Technique" for weight loss available on a website called http://www.mommystyle.com.

Tip #60: What to do after the lapse

It is a rare person who will not have a setback at some point during the journey toward a healthy eating lifestyle. The issue is not whether lapses occur, but the person's reaction. How can you learn to master those inevitable lapses? Here are six steps that can help.

1. *Stop, look, listen.* Stop what you are doing and examine the situation. What is occurring? Why are you lapsing? Be present in the moment. Consider moving yourself to a safe location where you won't be tempted and can think in a rational manner (take a walk, go to the gym, go to an open church, call a friend).

2. *Stay calm.* If you become anxious, the situation may get worse. You may conclude you are a hopeless binge eater and control is impossible. Pretend you are looking at yourself from a distance and ask what is going on over there. Separate yourself from the situation and view it as an objective observer. Forgive yourself and realize one lapse does not mean failure or immediate weight gain!

3. *Renew your weight loss vows.* Take a minute and remind yourself how far you have come, the progress you've made and how sad it would be to throw away all your hard work. Restart your goals, get determined and move ahead. Copy on an index card, and carry it with you when you need to renew your commitment

> **THERE IS NO OBSTACLE, NO SITUATION OR CIRCUMSTANCE THAT CAN CIRCUMVENT, HINDER, OR CONTROL THE FIRM RESOLVE OF A DETERMINED SOULD (LIKE ME) TO MAKE A CHANGE, FORM A HABIT, OR REACH A GOAL. I DO WHATEVER IT TAKES AND I KEEP ON WORKING UNTIL I AM SUCCESSFUL! I CAN! I WILL!**

4. *Analyze the situation.* Instead of blaming yourself and feeling guilty, use the situation as a learning experience. Do certain feelings,

places, activities (like TV watching), parties, restaurants put you at risk for bingeing? What will you do to defend yourself in the future and arm yourself with prevention?

5. ***Take charge immediately.*** Leap into action. Leave the house. Throw out the food. Turn off the TV. Take action without hesitation. Waiting is an excuse for letting go of control. Leave the environment and gain control faster.

6. ***Ask for help.*** Talk to your spouse, partner, friends, and co-workers. They can be surprisingly supportive if you are honest and tell them what you need.

Tip #61: Always know how many calories you need

Now that you've read this far and have determined you are ready to make the changes and necessary adjustments in your day-to-day life to accommodate fitness and healthy eating, it's time to be more specific about your eating program and take action.

This section is where you begin a new lifestyle, a new way of eating, and a new attitude about your body. From here on you will never be the same. You will have a body that you can be proud of and feel good about.

This tip, from my first book (The Fat to Muscle Challenge) and the *Eight Week Supplemental Program* (8-Week Miracle) are all step-by-step guides for decreasing body fat and adding muscle. Follow these suggestions and make continuous, slow, steady improvement for the rest of your life. Here's what you need to do. **First, determine your daily calorie needs. DO a metabolic profile** accurately and follow caloric intake guidelines on a regular, daily basis **WILL GUARANTEE A HEALTHY FAT LOSS AND BETTER BODY**. You will see a change in weight and a change in body fat composition in a much shorter period of time by creating your own METABOLIC PROFILE. What is a metabolic profile? A metabolic profile simply determines:

1. how many calories you burn during waking hours. The profile, also called a BMR includes the calories needed to maintain and sustain all your bodily functions such as heartbeat and digestion.

2. your calorie consumption based on lifestyle activities and exercise in the course of a day (accounts for 25 to 40% of your daily calorie consumption).

3. how many calories you need to consume on a daily basis to lose fat or add muscle mass and change the look of your body.

Jim Hart, A.C.E.

Weight loss is complicated and highly individualized. There are numerous diets, fitness gurus, pills, and gadgets that promise weight loss. Ultimately, losing weight all comes down to numbers. It's a simple equation: Calories in minus calories out.

To be successful, you must understand the equation and know your own numbers. Initially, you might resist the tedious task of keeping track of your calories, but if you don't do it for at least the first few weeks you probably won't lose weight. **The numbers don't lie**. <u>The figures provide you a more objective reality</u>.

Suppose you were saving money for a new car and on a whim decided to book a two-week luxury cruise to South America. When you're spouse asks how you can afford such a costly trip, you simply reply, "Not sure. I didn't have time to think it through. I forgot to look at the checking account statements, but I figured it will somehow all work out."

You come back from your trip and six months later you're still driving that old junker. Meanwhile, your credit card debt is up and the plumbing bill from the leak that ruined your carpets last month is looming over you. People think of spending calories in the same way. They make impulse choices about what to eat disregarding their weight loss goals or unaware of how the extra hidden calories in a restaurant meal will affect their body and its fat storage capacity.

Guessing and indiscriminate choices about food are two of the culprits in failed weight loss attempts. You need to have accurate calorie goal numbers and strive to meet them every day, making food choices that fit with your program.

The most important number in your daily plan is your basal metabolic rate (or BMR). The BMR is the calorie total that your body uses to perform basic functions like breathing and digesting food. 60 to 75% of your daily calories go towards these functions.

What you eat is called "Calories In" and the number your burn each day is "Calories Out." To lose weight, you need to consume fewer calories than your body requires.

<u>To determine that number, perform these calculations:</u>

USE THIS EQUATION

661 [**start with this figure**]
+   [4.38 **x** (your weight in pounds)]
+   [4.38 **x** (your height in inches)]
-    [4.7 **x** (your age)]
TOTAL = Your basal metabolic rate

An example for a 5'8" 42-year-old weighing 170 pounds:
661 [**initial starting point**]
+   [4.38 x 170 = 744.6]
+   [4.38 x 68 = 297.8]
-    (4.7 x 42 = 197.4)
TOTAL = 1,506.04

To figure your calories burned through activity, see the chart below. Multiply your BMR by the number that most accurately describes your activity level:

ACTIVITY LEVEL	MULTIPLIER
1. **Sedentary** – sitting, very little physical effort no manual labor, slow movement	**x 1.15**
2. **Light activity** – Doing normal, everyday tasks You spend most of your time at a desk or in a vehicle. You may walk from place to place but no more than 20 to 25 minutes per day. You may exercise or play sports occasionally, but no more than 90 minutes per week.	**x 1.3**
3. **Moderate** Your work involves some heavy lifting, operating Equipment, delivery work, cleaning, or otherwise physically demanding much of the time. You workout and exercise at least three times a week for an hour and work up a good sweat doing it.	**x 1.4**

4. **Very active**   **x 1.6**
You have a physically demanding occupation (construction work, landscaping, etc.) and you exercise or work up a good sweat at least 3-5 times a week for an hour or more each time

5. **Extremely active**   **x 1.8**
You are an amateur athlete or dedicated gym rat working Out or training vigorously 5-7 times a week for an hour or more. Your occupation is physically demanding (lumberjack, furniture mover, bicycle messenger).

Example: If you are extremely active, take your BMR and multiply by 1.8. Our previous gentleman had a BMR of 1,506.4. Multiplied by 1.8, the total calories this person burns is approximately 2,711/day.

On a daily basis, our example person's weight will remain the same if he eats 2,711 calories. To lose weight, he will need to decrease his calories or raise his activity level.

If you decrease your calories by 250 per week and increase your daily exercise activity to burn 1,750 calories a week (or 250 per day) you will lose one pound of fat per week. 500 calories per day X seven days = 3500, which is what is contained in a pound of fat.

Now, do your personal formulas here:
      661
+   [4.38 x (*insert your weight in pounds*_____)]
+   [4.38 x (*insert your height in inches*_____)]
-    [4.7 x (*insert your age in years*_____)]
_____ TOTAL = Your basal metabolic rate

NEXT
Multiply your BMR by one of the activity level multipliers from the chart. Your BMR = ____ X ____(*insert multiplier*) = _____ TOTAL calories you need to remain at your weight.

NOTE: To lose a pound of fat per week, reduce your daily calorie intake by 500 or exercise burning 250 more calories and reduce your food intake by 250 calories. A pound of fat is 3,500 calories. A 500 calorie reduction over 7 days = 3,500 less than BMR. Now, for those of you who moaned and groaned when you saw those equations, I have a faster shortcut. It's not as precise but it comes close and will give you a general range to strive for:

a. Multiply your weight by 10 if you have a slow metabolism and gain weight easily, regardless of how active or sedentary you are.

b. Multiply your weight by 12 if you are moderately active and have an average metabolism.

c. Multiply your weight by 15 if you have a physically demanding job, a fast metabolism (you don't gain weight easily, but if you do, it's usually in the abdominal region).

These calculations are for men over 40 who need to lose weight.

Example: If you work with computers all day, walk to work, garden on weekends, and gain weight easily after holidays or vacations, you have a slow metabolism. If you weighed 160 pounds you would multiply your weight by 12 and strive for a calorie count of 1,920 per day. It's okay to be a few hundred below or above that mark, the important thing is to **THINK WEEKLY**. At the end of the week, you should have consumed about 13,440 calories (7 x 1,920). Some days will be higher, some days lower, but it should come close to 13,440 by week's end. This allows you to have a few cheat meals and not feel guilty. If you go over by 500 calories at a Wednesday night restaurant meal, simply eliminate 83 calories (500 ÷ 6 = 83). From each of the six meals you consume on Thursday. It's simple! Just eliminate one apple, eat half the protein bar, or eat two less sweet potatoes and ½ a container of cottage cheese instead of an entire one. To lose a pound a week, reduce your daily calorie intake by 250 and burn 250 calories through exercise activity.

If you are still unsure how to figure your calories, use the *X Factor Way to Lose Fat*

X Factor	Fat weight to lose in pounds
14	0
13	1-5
12	6-10
11	11-15
10	16-20
9	over 20

Determine how much fat you want to lose. Multiply your current weight in pounds by the X Factor for your daily calorie needs. This is another excellent formula that has good accuracy.

Next step: keep a food journal

I know I've mentioned this several times, but I cannot stress enough how important this step really is. Write down everything you eat from breakfast to bedtime. This is one powerful and widely tested method for weight control success. It works if you do it! People who refuse to do this often consistently fail at their weight loss goals.

It may not be sexy, and you won't see any faded celebrities endorsing it, but a wealth of science and practical experience says keeping a food journal can help you lose weight, and, equally important, keep it off. In 1998, researchers from the Center for Behavioral Medicine and Sports Psychology in Chicago, IL, followed 38 dieters through the temptations of holiday eating. These men and women had already lost an average of twenty-one pounds during a 50-week weight-loss program. The 25% who religiously recorded every morsel that passed through their lips lost an average of seven pounds during the stretch of gluttony lasting from two weeks before Thanksgiving to two weeks after New Year's. The less diligent scribes gained back an average of three pounds (*Lifestyle Counselors Guide to Weight Control*, first edition).

This report, and others like it, led Daniel Kirschenbaum, Ph.D., director of the center and a member of the research team that carried out the study, to conclude in his book The 9 Truths about Weight Loss that "self monitoring is the single most important aspect of effective weight control."

A journal helps you with the following:

1. **Setting goals**. Goals are powerful motivators. If you set a goal of 30 fat grams a day, and every day you're counting fat grams, that motivates you, that encourages you. Monitoring is what makes goals come to life. You can say, "No more than 30 fat grams" but if you don't write it down and see whether you made it or not, it's just a vague thing. It is less likely that your plan will come to life.

2. **Making a commitment**. Once you get used to looking up fat grams, it takes maybe a minute per day. Every time you write something down it's like saying, "I believe it will help me; this matters in my life."

3. **Maintaining control.** Once you write it on paper, it takes the emotion out of the action. If you eat a donut and write it down, it doesn't have to become a Greek tragedy. It's just 12 fat grams.

4. **Providing information**. A journal helps you to be more aware of what you're eating, when you're eating, and how much you're eating. It's a great way to understand and diagnose what eating problems might transpire so you can start making changes.

Frequently Asked Questions

Question: I'm 62-years-old and walk about 1.5 miles per day and feel pretty good. I hear a lot about strength training for older adults but I'm not sure the efforts I need to make will really make any difference at my advanced age. What can I expect if I start lifting weights?

Answer: Here's an excellent article from exercise expert Wayne Westcott on the benefits of strength training for older adults (*Strength Training for Seniors: The Facts* accessed 8.30.2002 at healthy.net).

During the past several years, many studies have highlighted the health value of strength training for aging adults. Research at the University of Maryland has shown that strength training is effective for improving glucose metabolism, increasing bone mineral density, and speeding up gastrointestinal transit. Studies at Tufts University have demonstrated that strength exercise adds lean tissue, increases resting metabolism, and reduces arthritic discomfort. Extensive work at the University of Florida has shown that strength training increases low back strength and alleviates low back pain.

From an athletic perspective, research reveals that strength training improves golf performance by increasing club head speed and driving power. Empirical evidence indicates that strength exercise may also enhance other physical activities such as tennis and cycling.

While all of these health and performance factors are important, perhaps the most compelling concerns for most seniors are the three "B"s. These are bodyweight, body composition, and blood pressure. Generally speaking, senior men and women are concerned about gaining weight, getting soft, and experiencing elevated blood pressure. They have already discovered that dieting doesn't produce permanent weight loss, and that walking is not very effective for firming muscles. Quite true. They are afraid to try strength training because they've heard that it will increase their blood pressure. Untrue.

Several small-scale studies have shown that strength exercise is effective for decreasing bodyweight, increasing lean weight, and reducing resting blood pressure. In addition, strength training results in a higher resting metabolic rate and greater daily energy utilization.

But what specific change can seniors expect from a basic program of strength exercise? We recently analyzed data on 1,132 men and women who completed the South Shore YMCA basic fitness program. All of the participants performed 25 minutes of strength exercise and 25 minutes of endurance exercise, two or three days per week for a period of eight weeks.

The results of this relatively large research study should be encouraging news for senior men and women. Consider the following key findings for the 341 older adults who completed the eight-week basic fitness program.

1. Seniors can safely participate in a well-designed and carefully-supervised program of strength exercise. There were no injuries among the senior subjects in this study. Of course, all participants should have their physician's approval before beginning an exercise program.

2. Seniors can improve their body composition. The seniors in this exercise program reduced their percent fat by 2.0% after just two months of training. This was similar to the body composition improvements attained by the younger adults.

3. Seniors can decrease their fat weight. Like the younger program participants, the senior subjects lost more than four pounds of fat weight during the eight- week training period.

4. Seniors can increase their lean (muscle weight). The seniors in this study added 2.4 pounds of lean weight after two months of training. In the important area of muscle replacement, the senior men and women did just as well as the young and middle-aged adults.

5. Seniors can reduce their resting blood pressure. Following eight weeks of regular exercise, the senior subjects experienced a 3.7 mm Hg drop in their diastolic blood pressure. These resting blood pressure decreases were greater than those of the younger program participants.

6. Seniors can develop physically active lifestyles, even after years of sedentary behavior. Over 90 percent of the senior program participants continued to exercise after the completion of the study. They were highly satisfied with the results of the eight-

week exercise program and committed themselves to keep up their training efforts.

In summary, seniors have much to gain from regular strength training, particularly as part of a supervised exercise program. The senior men and women in this study reported looking, feeling, and functioning better, which is consistent with their recorded improvements in bodyweight, body composition, and resting blood pressure. It appears that an hour of exercise, two or three days a week is one of the best investments seniors can make for their health and fitness. (Wayne L. Westcott, Ph.D. is fitness research director at the South Shore YMCA in Quincy, MA and the author of the new Nautilus book, <u>Building</u> <u>Strength</u> <u>and</u> <u>Stamina</u>.)

Question: I'm hearing a lot about testosterone replacement for men over 40. Is it really worth the risk?

Answer: Testosterone builds muscle in older men. Muscle mass and usable muscle fibers drop by 20% between ages 40 and 60 (a condition known as sarcopenia). Things really go down hill from there. By age 70 to 80, some men are so debilitated that they have trouble moving effectively. What causes muscular decline in older men? Physical inactivity is the leading culprit, but decreased testosterone levels also play a role – dropping by 50% between ages 20 and 80. Dr. Virat Bakhski and colleagues from Virginia Commonwealth University, in Richmond, gave 15 elderly, debilitated men weekly injections of testosterone (100 mg.) for eight weeks. They found remarkable increases in muscle mass and strength that were comparable to gains from weight training. This study provides more evidence for the value of testosterone supplementation in older men. A big problem is that testosterone may increase the risk of prostate enlargement, prostate cancer, and coronary artery disease. But the results suggest giving testosterone to this population could improve quality of life (*Journal of American Geriatric Society*, Issue 48, 2000).

Question: My knees ache after my treadmill walking and my elbows and shoulders hurt and ache for several hours after I workout. Besides pain relievers are there any other natural products that can help relieve the aches and pains of an older athletic guy?

Answer: Here is a list of the top supplements that have been researched and show promised in relieving the minor aches and pains of overuse and minor rheumatoid arthritis:

1. A multivitamin containing selenium, manganese, zinc, niacin, and vitamins C & E;
2. gamma linolenic acid (good for arthritis);
3. MSM (helps with delayed onset muscle soreness and relieves the pain of rheumatoid arthritis); and,
4. the #1 most important product is GLUCOSAMINE. It is an actual component of connective tissue and cartilage. This substance plays a vital role in the formation of tendons, ligaments, and bones. It stimulates the manufacturing of chemicals that are necessary for joint repair and protects against further joint destruction.

Question: Jim, what is the best way to lose fat?

Answer: This is a complicated answer because there simply is no best way. However, there are some general guidelines that are universally proven to work for most people who make a good sustained effort.

Any activity that incorporates multiple muscle groups and weight bearing (e.g., strength training, circuit training, calisthenics, running, cycling, etc.) is ideal. It's a false assumption that low intensity exercise is best for fat loss. When exercising at a low intensity, the body uses a higher percentage of calories from fat. However, at a higher intensity, the number of calories used per minute is much greater and consequently the total number of fat calories great as well. The rate of energy used (as expressed in total calories) is more important when determining the exercise intensity that will use the most fat.

Endurance-trained runners and cyclists usually rely less on carbohydrates than fat as a fuel source. Therefore, the more aerobically trained you become, the higher amounts of fat you burn up during subsequent exercise sessions.

A little known fact is that you do not necessarily have to use fat during exercise. Much of the fat from adipose tissue (as opposed to intramuscular fat which is used during exercise) is lost in the hours following exercise. Moreover, the amount of fat lost after depends in part on the INTENSITY during the workout.

Following high intensity exercise, the rate of FAT OXIDATION is much higher than after low intensity exercise. Interval training is an ideal way to break up higher levels of intensity into more manageable segments. An example of interval training would be to jog at a moderate pace, then sprint for 30 seconds. This would be repeated six to 8 times over the course of a workout and dramatically helps to decrease body fat percentage.

A combination of endurance aerobic exercise and strength training has the greatest impact of fat loss than either regimen alone.

Question: How can I get that flat stomach and washboard abs?

Answer: Genetics, eating habits, and cardiovascular activity play a role in whether or not you can acquire the "six-pack." Having said that, two types of exercise can help strength training and cardiovascular exercise. The abs are just like any other muscle group; for their definition to become visible, they must grow larger and the fat that lies over them must decrease. What makes the definition of the abs so difficult is that they are situated in areas of the body that contains the most fat. So crunches are only half the story. You need to combine cardiovascular exercise with a reduction in calories to decrease body fat percentage to a point where you can see the abs. Most people don't do nearly enough cardio or reduce their calories enough to make any noticeable difference. Abs begin to miraculously appear when people do five intense 45 minute interval cardio sessions over a week and eat 10% less calories than they need for maintenance. Even quicker results are realized when the composition of the diet does not include sugar, flour, or heavy starchy foods.

Question: Should I do cardio first or weight train first?

Answer: It depends on your goal. There has been some debate about the theory that performing strength training before cardiovascular exercise will augment the amount of fat used during the cardio workout because strength training depletes the store of carbohydrates (muscle glycogen) and therefore the body will burn fat for fuel. Unfortunately, most people don't work at weightlifting intensely or long enough to deplete the sugar stores in the body because of the rest periods between sets. Even if you were able to deplete your glycogen stores completely, working in this state has many negative consequences including buildup of lactic acid, low blood insulin, hypoglycemia, and a fatigue described as "hitting a wall." Currently there is no scientific research that proves strength training before a cardio workout increases the amount of fat used.

The key to burning greater amounts fat is <u>INTENSITY OF ACTIVITY</u>, not the type of exercise. Do any activity with great intensity (sprint instead of jog, power lifting instead of machine exercise) and you will burn more fat stores. If your primary goal is to increase aerobic endurance or lose weight, <u>do cardio first</u>. If the primary goal is to increase strength and muscle mass, <u>weight train first</u>. Basically, to get the most out of the workout, you should do first what is most important. Since most people want to lose weight and increase muscle mass, the best thing to do is alternate the order of workouts during different cycles of training.

Question: What is my target heart rate?

Answer: Target heart rate is the measure used to determine the desired intensity of an activity. Using a heart rate monitor with a chest strap and a wrist watch receiver, you can get a fairly accurate analysis of how hard your heart pumps through various levels of exercise intensity. There are five zones of training intensity. The percentage in these zones is a number derived from determining an individual's maximum heart rate.

For years the standard formula utilized to determine your maximum heart rate was <u>220 – your age = max heart rate</u>. However, the formula does not take into account age or previously established fitness levels (i.e. seniors and athletes).

The new formula determined by testing 18,700 people at the National Institute of Health is as follows: 208 - .70 x (your age).

A follow-up study of 514 adults confirmed its power to accurately predict maximum heart rate. A 45-year-old man will have a maximum heart rate of 178.

<u>There are five zones of intensity that can be used for achieving your fitness goals</u>.

ZONE 1 *50 to 60% of max heart rate*

This zone is good for warm-ups and cool-downs, beginners, and seniors. This is the recovery zone for cool-down periods during intense interval training programs and for highly conditioned people and those who simply want to reduce risk of heart disease.

Walking, leisurely bike riding, gardening, and hiking fit into this category.

ZONE 2   *60 to 70% of maximum heart rate*
The next step on the fitness ladder, Zone2 includes mild forms of exercise for intermediate exercisers. Typical activities include vigorous walking, jogging, biking, EFX machines, aerobic classes, and light circuit weight training.

ZONE 3   *70 to 80% of maximum heart rate*
This is the true aerobic training zone used most frequently for endurance training, cardiovascular fitness, and weight loss. Running, rowing, calisthenics, high-intensity aerobic classes, and jumping rope are a few examples that will bring your heart rate into Zone 3.

ZONE 4   *80 to 90% of maximum heart rate*
Used by only the fittest trainees and athletes to improve performance for competition, Zone 4 is called the "lactate threshold zone" and creates fatigue in the legs and arms along with heavy breathing. This is where the body is on the edge of going into an anaerobic state. Sprinting, all out circuit weight training, stair running, and competition biking are sports that put the heart into zone 4.

ZONE 5   *90 to 100% of maximum heart rate*
The anaerobic zone is only achieved by the elite few. The body is using only glycogen and sugar for fuel. Zone 5 creates a lot of pain and is tolerable for a minute or so.

Question: How much exercise do I need to start seeing significant fat loss?

Answer: A study from the *Journal of the American Medical Association* looking at long-term weight loss in overweight adults using home exercise equipment came to the following conclusion:

> "At least 150 minutes of moderate exercise per week is necessary for weight loss and 200 or more is required for significant weight loss. Two hundred minutes is equivalent to 1,500 to 2,000 calories expended per week. Moderate exercise increases the heart rate up to 70%/80% of maximum predicted heart rate."

A new study from the University of Wisconsin showed that day-long fat use was higher when subjects exercised intensely for shorter periods of time (20-30 minutes of interval training) rather than moderately for 40 to 50 minutes, although increased fat loss was seen in individuals performing moderate exercise five days a week for 45 minutes.

Question: Should I hire a personal trainer?

Answer: Yes! A new study found that supervised exercisers showed greater increases in strength, and that those strength increases occurred more rapidly in supervised exercisers than they did in non-supervised exercisers. The 12-week study, which recently was published in *Medicine and Science in Sports and Exercise*, involved 20 men ages 18 to 35. They all had a year or two of experience with resistance training, but none of them had ever worked with a personal trainer.

By the end of the study, significant strength gains were achieved by both groups. However, fat-free mass increased with significance only in the supervised group. Also, the supervised group showed greater increases in strength, and made those strength gains at a quicker rate than the other group. The men in the supervised group showed a 30- to 45-percent higher improvement in maximal strength than the unsupervised group.

Researchers concluded that the use of greater training loads, plus immeasurable factors such as competitiveness and external motivation all may have contributed to the greater gains made by the supervised group. Whatever the reasons, according to this study, the assistance of a trainer can help maximize fitness results in a faster time.

Question: Do fat burners work?

Answer: No "fat burner" is going to cut that dirty dozen unless you control your calorie intake and train with weights three or four times a week. Now, if you're already doing that, here's the next step: start doing aerobic exercise three or four times a week. Begin with 20 minutes at a moderate intensity level (pulse rate around 120 to 140 beats per minute) and then add one more minute of aerobic exercise, every other day, until you hit 40 minutes, then don't go beyond that.

Now, I strongly believe the best time to do aerobics is as soon as you get up in the morning on an empty stomach. If you want to get even better fat-burning results from that exercise, try using a fat burner like the TwinLab's Ripped Fuel, or Neo Elite Nutrition's new Phen-Free about 30 minutes before you do your morning aerobics. These burners help "liberate" stored body fat to be used as fuel during aerobic exercise.

Question: Should I strive for a certain percentage of protein, fat, and carbohydrates? What about those diets that stress ratios of 40-40-30 with high fats, low carbs?

Answer: From years of training and nutrition coaching, I have rarely seen a person who can consistently know the percentage they acquire with every meal. I try not to get too stringent with percentage numbers because I prefer to emphasize eating and enjoying a wide variety of foods, with moderation over a range of calories that works for each individual. I recommend staying within your calorie range as the top priority. The second priority is to watch the fat grams per meal. I am still a believer in the theory that fats turn to fat faster than carbs or protein. Fats have twice the calorie density and require almost no energy from your body for breakdown. Protein and carbs are more complex and require a longer period to be metabolized. In fact, 25% of the calories you consume in protein or carbs goes toward digestion. So, a 100 calorie chicken breast is giving your body 75 calories, whereas a 100 calorie pat of butter translates to 100 calories for your body to use or store as fat.

A simple rule regarding fat intake:

If your calorie base is: Then take in this amount of fat grams/day:
(This should be 20% of your overall daily intake)

1,800	40-50 grams/day
2,000	40-50 grams/day
2,200	40-50 grams/day
2,400	52-62 grams/day
2,600	52-62 grams/day
2,800	52-62 grams/day

Always go for good fat sources like nuts, fish oils (from salmon and fatty fish), olive oil, flaxseed, and natural oils found in vegetables (broccoli) and grains (oatmeal, wheat germ). Avoid saturated palm, coconut, lard, or hydrogenated oils found in most processed foods and fast food.

As for protein, I recommend a wide range based on your activity level and calorie range. A good rule for most people is 1.0 to 1.5 grams per pound of body weight each day. For example, a 160 lb. man would need between 160-240 (160 x 1.0 and 160 x 1.5) grams of protein per day. At each meal, it's a wise plan for one to strive for 26 to 40 grams of protein. A small chicken breast, a 12-ounce container of cottage cheese, or a can of tuna fish will come within that range.

Carbohydrates are a source of controversy with today's high-fat, high-protein diet craze. If you are eating mostly fibrous carbohydrates like vegetables, salad greens, garbanzo beans, fresh fruit and sweet potatoes, you can usually avoid worry about counting calories or carbo-grams. However, consuming high starch carbohydrates (which can be a good source of energy if used in moderation) like pasta, bread, rice, white potatoes, cereals, and most processed foods including protein bars, can be tricky depending on how well your body handles them. Some people do well while eating bread, pasta, and sugar-filled products while others only begin to see a reduction in body fat when they reduce or eliminate these items.

Here are some guidelines—

If your calorie range is: You should strive for a daily carb intake of:

1,800	180 grams
2,000	200 grams
2,200	220 grams
2,400	240 grams
2,600	260 grams
2,800	280 grams

Divide six meals per day to get your carbs per meal (i.e. 2,800 calories = 280 grams of carbohydrates ÷ 6 meals/day = 46.6 grams of carbohydrates/ meal).

Here are some suggestions for visually mastering portion control when there is no scale or measuring cups to help. You can cure ***portion distortion*** with imagery. Picture:

- Three ounces of meat, poultry, or fish are about the size of one deck of playing cards or the palm of a woman's hand.
- A computer mouse is the size as a medium potato
- One-half cup of cut fruit or vegetables, pasta, or rice is about the size of a small fist
- One cup of milk, yogurt, or chopped fresh greens is about the size of a small hand holding a tennis ball
- One ounce of cheese is about the size of your thumb
- Two tablespoons of peanut butter is no larger than the size of a golf ball
- 1 pancake or waffle serving should be about the diameter of an audio CD
- Single serving of fruit, rice, or vegetables is about the size of a tennis ball
- A softball sized serving of pasta is near 3 ounces
- 8 ounce fish serving is about the size of a videocassette (tuna, salmon)

Why eat six times per day? New research indicates that energy deficits of only hours, not days, appear to set the body up to retain fat. A number of recent studies have associated dietary restrictions or poor time eating with such unwanted changes as lower metabolism, higher body fat, higher injury rates, menstrual dysfunction, and reduced bone density (WebMD Health BMI "Spotting Fad Diets," http://www.webmd.com/content/article/2731.1647).

Now begin reading the *"Eight Week Miracle Plan for Cardiovascular Exercise and Strength Training"* and use tools that will move you towards having the body and lifestyle you've been wishing and dreaming about! Good luck!

Weight Loss Profiles

Perry Monastero

Height: 5'6"
Age: 33
Starting weight: 165; Body Fat: approximately 20%
Current weight: 140; Body Fat: approximately 9%
Months/years at current goal weight/fitness level: 2.5

Daily eating plan: Several small meals per day and usually makes a point to eat lots of protein, veggies, and fruits. Client avoids sugar, most alcohol, most starches, and limits processed foods.

Exercise routine: five times/week (plays soccer at least once a week; weight trains about three to four times per week)

Question: What was your turning point?

Answer: I was frustrated from not losing fat after years of exercising. I was running vigorously five times/week and playing soccer and biking everywhere, exercising altogether 5 hours/week. A friend suggested I see a nutritionist. He nudged me, saying my problem was probably caused by my diet. I was referred to Jim and the rest is history. Turns out my friend was right. I didn't realize I was eating a disproportionate amount of unhealthy foods. Jim taught me about food and how to eat more healthfully. Additionally, Jim encouraged me to build the confidence to strength training a try.

Barnett J. Jarman

Height: 5'11"; Starting Weight: 154; Current Weight: 168
Months at current goal weight: 1.5
Daily eating plan: Breakfast – two eggs; 2 slices of toast; hash browns, coffee, water, OJ
　　　　Snack – ProMax protein bar

Lunch – 1 can of tuna with bagel and chips
Snack – Promax protein bar
Dinner – ½ cup of rice, black beans, chicken breast

Exercise routine: Strength trains 4-5 times/week for 1 to 1.5 hours each

"I got started because my partner gave me four sessions with Jim. The turning point took place in August 2001 when I had bulked up, gained 8 pounds, and developed good muscle tone. The biggest reward was that I felt good about my well-being and pleased with how I looked physically."

Question: How have you been able to stick with it? How do you deal with everyday temptations, temporary setbacks, and lapses?

Answer: "I have reached a point where I really enjoy working out; however, from time to time, I encounter setbacks with my health that slows me down and also alters my eating. I generally start back slowly and build back up to my routines."

Question: What changes or sacrifices have you made to your daily life schedule to make fitness and eating right a priority?

Answer: "I have continuously altered my eating to include more protein (chicken breasts, ProMax boars, protein shakes, etc.). I have also progressed from 1-2 workouts monthly to four to five times/week over the past year. I have also begun to take a supplement called L-Glutamine."

Question: What is the biggest reward for you in reaching and maintaining your fitness and eating lifestyle?

Answer: "The biggest reward for me is how well I feel from my workouts both physically and mentally."

Question: What advice would you give to others who are starting out?

Answer: "I would say to start slow and to set realistic goals, understand your body, and know where to push and not to push. Have fun – it can become a way of life."

Vaughn Cook

Months/years at current goal weight: 5 years

Daily Eating Plan: "I try to eat five to six smaller meals per day with a constant check on calories, fat, carbohydrates, and protein content.

I basically have three breakfast meals that I alternate. Egg white omelettes and oatmeal, strawberries with non-fat cottage cheese and oatmeal or Keto cereal and high-protein, low-carb pancakes with either oatmeal or Keto cereal. I now have a third choice of a new breakfast frozen entrée with low carbs and high protein.

In between meals are usually protein bars or Dannon yogurt with Fat Free Cool Whip or something similar along with fruit.

Lunch varies with salads and soup to wraps and soup to low calorie high protein frozen entrée's such as Lean Cuisine.

Dinner at home is usually chicken or fish with frozen vegetables and salad or sweet potato. Dinner out is scrutinized, as much as possible, for how food is cooked and content."

Exercise Routine: "I workout with Jim Hart twice a week. I also do cardio on off days by way of the EFX machine; in warmer months, lots of biking. Sometimes I do a workout on my own.

Our workouts vary from routine machine exercises to new and innovative workouts developed by Jim through his constant attendance at seminars and reading. One of the worst things that used to happen to me was that I would get bored with my workout routine and then have yet another excuse not to go to the gym."

Question: How did you get started? What was your turning point? What motivated you? What is the biggest reward for having achieved your goals?

Answer: I got started working out when I was in my early thirties but never had a workout plan so I got varying results. It was very easy to skip workouts for many reasons. I worked out with various partners over the years which helped in getting me to the gym, but again no real program to follow. Hit and miss routines. My turning point was when I started working out with Jim Hart five years ago. He is a professional who gives me both the support and discipline that I need to maintain a healthy body and good diet.

My motivation was in seeing Jim working with others and he seemed to have more to offer than some trainers whom I had watched over a period of time. The big plus was that when I began talking to Jim, I found out just how well versed he is in the whole body and mind, not just in muscles.

The biggest reward for having achieved my goals, although I have other goals to achieve, is the knowledge that my mind, body, self-esteem and health have been elevated to a degree that I'm sure that I couldn't have achieved on my own.

Question: How have you been able to stick with it? How do you deal with everyday temptations, temporary setbacks, and lapses?

Answer: I believe that I have been able to stick with the exercise and diet by virtue of the fact that I can have a day to cheat, if I care to, and not feel guilty. As long as I go back to my program the very next day, I will be OK. The way I ward off daily temptations is to be sure that I eat my five to six small meals per day so that when I run across cookies, potato chips, or ice cream, that I am not that hungry, so I can more easily say "no."

Being human, I have had lapses especially on vacation. But my routine has trained me to allow myself that occasional slip and to get right back on the beam."

Question: What changes or sacrifices have you made to your daily life schedule to make fitness and eating right a priority?

Answer: "One change was that I would eat more often and working from my home makes that easier. I have, however, envisioned myself in an office work situation. I know that I would prepare meals to take to work the night before. I have done this when visiting friends whom I know have no healthy food in their home. Another change is that I will now cook at home more often than I ever did.

Sacrifices? I don't know that I have made many. To consider going to the gym instead of, for instance, going to a mall or a movie or eating a fat diet now seems to be a very easy decision. By working out, I feel I have more energy to do many of the things that I like to do."

Question: What advice would you give to others that are starting out?

Answer: Don't think that you can't afford to have a trainer or to eat healthy. When I consider how much money I would spend and have spent on other things, a trainer, and the results you get far outweigh the cost. I know that I have idle time, I can spend a lot of money on items that I really don't need. This time can be better spent working on your body and mind. A salad is much cheaper than a big Mac.

Eating healthy can be expensive, but doesn't have to be. It's your choice. Many of my friends have said that they can't afford to eat healthy and they don't want to eat "blue milk and twigs." I have shown them that they can eat healthy for less. One way is by following the advice and recipes in the book "Fat to Muscle Challenge," by Jim Hart. Using everyday foods that you can purchase in any supermarket, these recipes give you easy AND fast meal plans with every step of the way instruction.

Lastly, don't be intimated by others in the gym. I always say that people at the gym don't have time to look at you because they are too busy looking at themselves in the mirror.

Steve Weixler

Months/years at current goal weight or desired level of fitness: 2

Daily eating plan: "I choose the maximum protein, moderate carbs and minimum fat possible in each menu. I try to eat smaller meals rather than larger. Since a highly structured home-prepared diet is not emotionally or practically possible for me, I always look at a menu or shop in the market for the freshest and lowest fat foods. When I absolutely have to cheat, I do. I have never completely given up a favorite food or beverage."

Exercise routine: "I have two separate workouts, once a week with Jim Hart. Once a week I go by myself."

Question: How did you get started? What was your turning point? What motivated you? What is the biggest reward for having achieved your goals?

Answer: I started to get a fresh workout routine to do by myself. Then, I transitioned to twice a week with Jim. The turning point was committing to scheduled workouts. My motivation was initially to lose body fat and to gain muscle mass. The biggest reward is the feeling of fitness and the sense that I'm taking care of myself the best way possible.

Question: How have you been able to stick with it? How do you deal with everyday temptations, temporary setbacks, and lapses?

Answer: I stick with it through the knowledge that each workout is an incremental step to the goal. If I miss one of eat the wrong things, I go back to the routine as soon as possible. I don't punish myself for lapses, but get back to the routine.

Question: What changes or sacrifices have you made to your daily life schedule to make fitness and eating right a priority?

Jim Hart, A.C.E.

Answer: I started to think about what I was eating. I learned to ration comfort food and make other substitutions for rewards. I made a deliberate, consistent time commitment and notified others in my life about it.

Question: What is the biggest reward for you in reaching and maintaining your fitness and eating lifestyle?

Answer: Looking and feeling well.

Question: What advice would you give to others who are starting out?

Answer: Make a long-term commitment to diet and exercise. Don't let yourself worry about how your body and appearance compares to others. Work with a trainer on a regular basis: if not ever week, at least monthly. Set realistic weight/body fat goals—but set them. As soon as you can see some progress, buy an attractive new item of clothing and wear it.

Mike Treat

Daily Eating Plan: "Previously (i.e. before I joined the HartBody plan), my diet had a large portion of carbohydrates in contrast to protein and fat. Since I enjoy running, this diet was OK. I also ate two meals per day. I was lucky to get in 1,500 calories per day. I wanted to gain more lean body mass and build up my upper body which was not in proportion to my lower body. After joining Hartbody, I was educated on the correct way to eat – six meals per day at 400 calories/meal (my situation) on average. Additionally, I found it very difficult to consume over 2,000 calories (not to mention 2,400 which is my optimal intake for my metabolism). In time (about three months) I got used to it and I started to switch to a higher protein diet which significantly helped me build up lean upper body mass. To get to this point took me about six months. I currently eat around five (sometimes six) small meals per day with an average of 55% protein, 30/35% carbohydrates and the balance, fat. I need to get back to a more consistent daily diet plan and to be stricter on all of this."

Exercise routine: "Since running is my favorite sport and since I have been doing this since I was in my teens, I make sure I get in my weekly miles which is about 30 miles on average. My goal is to go up to 40 miles per week. I am currently running 35 miles/week with a long run on Sunday, which is no more than 12 miles. My mile pace for long runs is between 9:00 and 9:30. The balance of my other runs is around 8:00 pace. My Vo2Max is at 60 with a max HR at 178. My lactic acid threshold (anaerobic threshold) is around 162 BPM.

Now that I started resistance training, I really enjoy it very much since I can see results and I notice that it is helping me in my running (both in form and in speed). I normally do resistance training for about 50 minutes every other day per instructions for the specific set(s) that I am doing. The challenging part is to balance or merge this type of training with my endurance training on those days, which I have to do both back-to-back (without overdoing and making myself prone to injury/infection). I take my morning heart rate every day (before I wake up) to make sure I can minimize any over training that I may be doing. This will help me to prevent or minimize injury in future routines (endurance or resistance routines).

I used to incorporate stretching (flexibility training) into my daily routine for about 30 minutes every day. I am now starting to get back to this since this is a major preventative to injury."

Question: How did you get started? What was your turning point? What motivated you? What is the biggest reward for having achieved your goals?

Answer: I always wanted to get more of an upper body so that started me to look around for a personal trainer since I did not want to do this without expert guidance since I heard and seen many of my friends who hurt themselves by lack of guidance. Since I was already a member of the 12th Street Gym, I thought it would make sense to get resistance training lessons there in concert with my aerobic training, which I was doing in the Cardio room. There was no major turning point for me. I just did it.

The biggest reward for me is when my friends (who did not see me for about 6 – 8 months) noticed the firmer shape I had and the build-up of my upper body which I never had before. In addition to this, the other part of this (which is just as important, if not more) is that resistance training has a lot of beneficial health factors associated to it. Additionally, this coupled with endurance training provides synergistic effects that are obvious in a physical, mental/spiritual and overall health aspects.

Question: How have you been able to stick with it? How do you deal with everyday temptations, temporary setbacks, and lapses?

Answer: The determination to get to my goals is the way I do this. I do this even with my work and most activities in my personal life. Some of my friends would personify me to a Mack Truck, "When Mike moves on something there is no stopping his momentum from getting what he wants." I think this is true in my life. Sure, I have setbacks and lapses, but I cope with them. A few of them are health issues (like being sick with the flu) and in these incidences, one cannot do much about them except to rest and get better. I stick with it [training] since I always want to improve and learn more. By entering into organized races is a goal that will make me stick to training besides the goal of improved health and personal appearance. I do listen to my body and at times, I will stop my routines if I feel something is not correct since I do not want that to propagate itself to even a more significant issue which can cause major injury. If I have a setback, I may be frustrated since I hate to start from square one and go through all the pains and effort to attain where I previously left off. Not much one can do (you just have to pick up your bags and move on).

Question: What changes or sacrifices have you made to your daily life schedule to make fitness and eating right a priority?

Answer: This was a tough one for me (especially the eating changes). It was hard for me to eat six meals per day and to get up to 2,400 calories per day. I did it, but I can still improve on it. Some of the changes were that I now have a storage cabinet in my office which contains tuna, protein bars, Myoplex drink packages, and an electric hand blender. In addition to that, I store perishable foods in the fridge at work (like fat-free cheese,

Myoplex pre-made drinks, and yogurt). I also am purchasing high protein foodstuffs for home as well. I eat less pasta and luckily my mother cannot cook as much like she used to due to her health. I am eating a lot more red meat as well (I was lucky if I ate a big steak once a month when I was on a more carb diet). I now eat red meat once a week (albeit it is loaded with saturated fat and cholesterol), I think my 35 miles per wekk will minimize the impact of this on my cardiovascular system by promoting higher HDL levels and minimizing LDL and VLDL levels). I believe that health is the most important "thing" we have in our life and therefore it should be the top priority for us. I still cheat once in a while and I still have a few beers with my friens every week. I do believe in a balanced lifestyle and not focused on one thing since this can be an end to everything (in fact, it can lead to terminating friendships when you have no time for your friends due to your focus on your training "requirements").

Question: What is the biggest reward for you in reaching and maintaining your fitness and eating lifestyle?

Answer: I think there are two for me. Health and overall physical appearance. Health is numero uno!

Question: What advice would you give to others who are starting out?

Answer: Have patience, stick with it, don't get discouraged if you have a lapse or setback (just pick up your bags and move on) and make sure that you have fun while doing it. Attitude is very important. I would also say that one should "listen" to his/her body. If you feel something is not just right, then stop and analyze what is happening before it's too late. Don't try to take on too much at once (I know, I did this and I got hurt which required an epidural shot in my neck).

Dominic Wolocko

Starting weight: 190#; Body fat: 29%
Current weight: 165#; Body fat: 17%
Years at current goal weight: 1.5 years

Daily eating plan: six small meals per day (high protein, low fat); one day of eating anything; supplements: protein powder and creatine

Exercise routine: Weights three times per week; cardio three times per week

Question: How did you get started? What was your turning point? What motivated you? What is the biggest reward for having achieved your goals?

Answer: I felt overweight, sluggish, and saw a rise in my blood pressure. I wanted to change my metabolism and gain energy in order to renovate the old house that I had bought. The biggest reward was losing the weight and toning my body and feeling and looking better at 46 than at 26 or 36. I went from 33" pants to wearing a 30"!

Question: How have you been able to stick with it? How do you deal with everyday temptations, temporary setbacks, and lapses?

Answer: Occasionally, I feel it's all right to have a setback, but no matter what, one must continue to begin again and keep up with the program. Once the metabolism changes, I find it maintains itself as far as weight goes.

Question: What changes or sacrifices have you made to your daily life schedule to make fitness and eating right a priority?

Answer: I avoid fast food and vendors and try to exercise at the beginning of my day – that helps to maintain and motivates me throughout the day. Also, trying to get more than 7 hours of sleep each day.

Question: What is the biggest reward for you in reaching and maintaining your fitness and eating lifestyle?

Answer: Energy and a new sense of self-esteem while aging.

Question: What advice would you give to others who are starting out?

Answer: Get through the first 12 weeks and you will definitely see and feel a change in yourself and then it becomes much easier to keep going.

Paul Parrott

Height: 5'11"
Starting weight: 253#
Current weight: 205#
Years at this fitness level: about one year
Exercise routine: strength training twice a week; cardio twice per week

Question: What is your daily eating plan?

Answer: I eat a good breakfast. Then, a snack followed by a balanced lunch and dinner. I try to keep my calories to about 2,800. My fat intake I try and keep at 15% of my total caloric intake.

Question: How did you get started? What was your turning point? What motivated you? What is the biggest reward for having achieved your goals?

Answer: Hiring Jim Hart got me started. I had tried various "diets" and exercise programs before, but they n ever stuck. Jim had the correct motivation techniques to keep me going. The fact that I feel better physically and mentally is my biggest reward.

Question: How have you been able to stick with it? How do you deal with everyday temptations, temporary setbacks, and lapses?

Answer: For the most part, yes. The most important and totally new way I deal with temptations is that if I do have a setback I don't feel as though I ruined it all and give up. Jim has proven to me that a small setback is not important and will happen and not to put too much importance in it.

Question: What changes or sacrifices have you made to your daily life schedule to make fitness and eating right a priority?

Answer: Probably finding the time to exercise.

Question: What advice would you give to others who are starting out?

Answer: Make up your mind and just stick to it. Give it a chance and you'll see it's not out of reach – even for somebody who has never been a "gym person" or fitness fanatic.

Web Resources

General Fitness Information:

T-Mag.com – general information on bodybuilding and supplements
Global-fitness.com
GymAmerica.com – online training and support
Mensfitness.com
Fitnessonline.com
Enutrition.com
PTonthenet.com – good articles on exercise nutrition and general fitness

Supplement Information:

Supplementinfo.org – consumer advocacy site on all types of supplements
Consumerlab.com
AnabolicReview.com
Steroid-Encyclopedia.com – information on steroids

Nutrition Information:

Ediets.com – do-it-yourself eating program
Cyberdiets.com – another do-it-yourself eating program
Dietstogo.com – food delivery service
EatRight.org – find a dietitian – American Dietetic Association-sponsored site
In2Nutrition.com – personalized nutrition and exercise programs
VirtualNutritionist.com
Diet-Coaching.com
EatWize.com – customized nutrition plans
PoundsAweigh.com

Health/Food Services:

Exoticmeats.com (800-680-4375)
888eatgame.com – your source for super-lean game meats
Melissas.com – "World's best exotic produce."
AST-ss.com – supplement and vitamin resource
DMOZ.org/shopping/food/diet – find sugar-free/fat-free/low-carb products

SugarFreeKitchen.com – Resource for low-carb, low sugar foods
SugarFreeMarket.com – same as above
FatFreeFoods.com
PizzaFree.com – high protein, low-fat pizza
SugarFreeParadise.com – low-carb breads & baked goods
Netrition.com – offers food products, bodybuilding supplements, and vitamins
Synergydiet.com – good selection of sugar jams, baked goods, and sweets
Robinsnest.org – Great selection of sugar-free, fat-free cakes

Inspiration & Motivation:

Worldpeakperformance.com – inspirational motivation and coaching
PoundsAWeigh.com – Daily inspiration for healthy living
TheWinningMind.com – improve mental fitness to enhance your sport/workout
Fitnessfind.com/justdoit.html – motivational articles to keep you motivated

Treating injuries:

Deroyal.com/shop – healthcare kits for treating foot problems and sports injuries SportsInjuryClinic.net

Mature Adult Fitness:

FitnessAge.com – An assessment tool that compares your chronological age to your body's true age based on your level of fitness, lifestyle, and habits
TGCMagazine.com – Fitness after 50
MyPrimeTime.com – lifestyle, health/fitness for the Baby Boomer generation
ICAA.CC – International Council on Active Aging
Healthy.net (Health World Online for Mature Adult)
Sandowmuseum.com/ironstargym – bodybuilding site for men over 40
ExerciseGroup.com/Fitnessafter40

Miscellaneous:

Tupperware.com – Best containers for packing healthy meals

Hartbody, Inc.

I always provide tailored recommendations for my clients' fitness and nutrition. Please complete the form to receive specific information related to your needs. Thanks!

Name: _____

Street Address: _____

City, State, Zip: _____

Phone numbers—Day: (   ) —   Night: (   ) —

Email address: _____@_____

Please circle one response for each question:

Do you want to learn more about how to eat when traveling?
                                                    YES   NO

Do you need information on vitamins, minerals and supplements?
                                                    YES   NO

Would you like to learn more about massage?   YES   NO

Have you any questions about fitness training or weight training?
                                                    YES   NO

Are you curious to learn how to eat more but gain less weight?
                                                    YES   NO

Want to learn about my personal coaching services? YES   NO

Jim Hart, A.C.E.

In what other areas are you interested in improving yourself?

_____

_____

_____

_____

Dear Reader:

First and foremost, I feel I must both congratulate and recognize my clients for whom this book is dedicated. It is through their determination to live a healthier, happier, and more fulfilling life that I was duly inspired to write this book. Thank you all for your support and encouragement!

My best regards in good health and fitness,

Jim

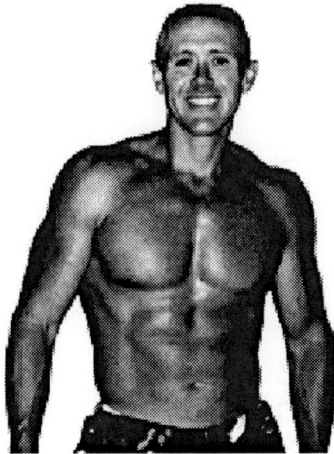

Jim Hart, A.C.E.

About the Author

Born in 1960, Jim Hart is a Philadelphia native who resides and works in Center City at the 12th Street Gym. A former grocery store manager, Hart is currently in this twelfth year as a personal trainer with certifications from the American Council on Exercise (A.C.E.) and the University of Pennsylvania Lifestyle and Nutrition Management program. Hart has over two decades' experience in strength training along with certifications in nutrition and eating/food disorders consulting. Hart earned a B.A. degree from LaSalle University in communication and is a master chef graduate from The Restaurant School (Philadelphia, Pennsylvania). A former corporate catering entrepreneur, Jim authored his first book The Fat to Muscle Challenge in 1999, a guide to eating well and losing weight.

Jim gives seminars and cooking demonstrations on enjoying the pleasures of healthy, nutritious foods. He creates fitness and eating plans that fit each individual client's lifestyle. Jim enables his clients to reach their goals to live happier, healthier lives. Jim is passionate about all aspects of fitness and integrates fun, competition, and challenge into all of his programs. Jim Hart has competed in bodybuilding competitions for masters and has run competitively in 5K races and half-marathons. Jim is also a certified massage therapist.

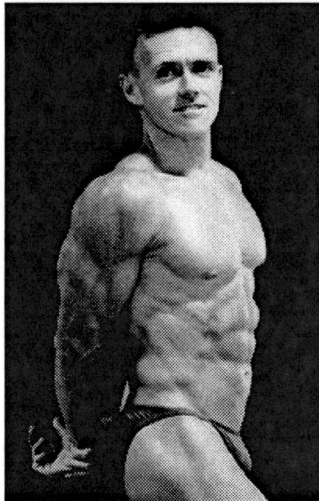

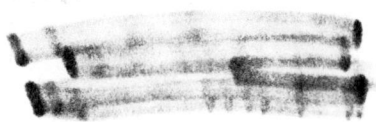

DATE DUE

CPSIA information can be obtained at www.ICGtesting.com
Printed in the USA
LVOW061744061211

258108LV00005B/136/A

9 781418 441548